ROB PARR'S

Post-Pregnancy Workout

"Rob Parr has shaped up what are, quite simply, some of the best bodies in Hollywood. The firm, fit form that served as a canvas for Demi Moore's painted-on suit on *Vanity Fair*'s cover was a Parr masterpiece. Likewise Madonna's strong, sculpted look and rock-star stamina."
—*Longevity*

"On the seventh day, God created Rob Parr."
—Liz Rosenberg, Madonna's publicist, *USA Today*

"His clients both look and perform like athletes; they are conditioned enough to play almost any sport."
—*Vogue*

"Rob Parr has run around the world with Madonna and helped Demi Moore get ready for maximum exposure in *Indecent Proposal*."
—*Shape*

"Madonna's fitness secret is Rob Parr, a former baseball player with a crooked grin and a degree in exercise physiology."
—*Cosmopolitan*

"I've worked with Rob for some time now and have found that a lot more women are noticing me. Unfortunately, my wife also works out with Rob. Tsk."
—James Caan

ROB PARR'S
Post-Pregnancy Workout

Rob Parr and
David A. Rudnitsky

Berkley Books, *New York*

ROB PARR'S POST-PREGNANCY WORKOUT

A Berkley Book / published by arrangement with
the authors

PRINTING HISTORY
Berkley trade paperback edition / January 1997

The Putnam Berkley World Wide Web site address is http://www.berkley.com/berkley

ISBN: 0-425-15607-9

BERKLEY®
Berkley Books are published by The Berkley Publishing Group,
200 Madison Avenue, New York, New York 10016.
BERKLEY and the "B" design
are trademarks belonging to Berkley Publishing Corporation.

PRINTED IN THE UNITED STATES OF AMERICA

10   9   8   7   6   5   4   3   2   1

With love I dedicate this book to my wife, Debra, and our wonderful children, Jordan, Hunter, and Chandler
—ROB PARR

To John and Barbara Jordan who are always there, and always care
—DAVID A. RUDNITSKY

Acknowledgments

Many thanks to all the people who helped me put this book together, especially all of my clients for the past fifteen years. A very special thanks to Demi Moore, Maria Shriver, Tatum O'Neal, Patti Scialfa and Theresa Russell, for trusting me during their pregnancies and post-pregnancies. I would also like to thank Madonna for the exposure and opportunities that our four-year collaboration offered me. Many thanks to David Rudnitsky and Rob Cohen for helping to make this book possible.

—Rob Parr

To Rob Cohen for starting the gestation process; to Denise Silvestro for guiding this book from inception through birth; to Lynn Bregman Blass and Jacob Blass for raising a true miracle named Zackers; to Allen Lissauer for executive-producing two great girls; to Genevieve Shapiro for nurturing Barry's inner child; to Barbara Jane Schwartz and Jerry Flum for combining their genes just perfectly; to Steve and Wendy Hans for creating Matthew and Dylan.

To Nancy and Dave Harding and their little Hardette, Nathaniel Cross; to Diane and Larry Lantz, who get quite a workout with Craig; to Sami Silverberg for making sure the family goes one more generation; to Eve Brandstein for birthing great ideas and raising a great kid named Benjamin; to Elayne Kahn; to Erica Ress for nursing so many ideas from infancy.

To Nancy Kitchen for having a child of Tiffany quality; to Arnie and Rachel Mann for moving and still grooving; to Grace and Bill Larsen for their enduring friendship and support; to Helen Uffner for just being the fabulous woman she is; to Helen Lynch for providing a home away from home; to Elyss Emmer for her incredible style and sparkle; to Spike and

Debbie Sorrentino, who are batting an incredible three for three; to Steve and Janet Klaussner for bringing forth Alexandra the Great; to Toni Attel for being a truly wonderful mother—in a past life.

To Florence Feuerman, without whom there'd be no Kenny; to Jim and Maddy Zimring for generously opening their hearts and home; to Joyce Ferman for having the enthusiasm of a child; to Lillian Levitt for her boundless love beyond the call of duty; to Mary Weinberg, nationally acclaimed co-author of Barbara; to Paul and Paulette Cooper, the proud parents of two furry four-legged children; to Paula Paizes and Richard Gonda for being part of the "King's Road" family; to Suzanne Lopez, who crossed time and space to find her true daughter, Anjelica Chiavani; to Skip and Ann Martin and of course Sylvia Novak for their friendship through trials of fire; and finally, to Mrs. Mollie Rudnitsky, who continues to have a great figure, even forty-five years after pregnancy.

—David A. Rudnitsky

Contents

The Post-Pregnancy Training

Practically everyone remembers the photo of a pregnant Demi Moore on the cover of *Vanity Fair*. Widely acclaimed, it was a stunning portrait that virtually revolutionized the image of expectant women across the country. Of course, it also generated a lot of controversy in the process. But there's never been any controversy about how Demi has gloriously regained, and continues to maintain, her world-class figure and star status.

And who in the world hasn't heard about the controversy that swirls around Madonna wherever she goes and whatever she does? But there's absolutely no controversy about her incredible stamina and physical appeal, the way in which she's managed to stay in peak condition for well over a decade of grueling performances.

Both of these women have made a commitment to shaping, reshaping, and indeed transforming their bodies. But I guarantee, there's nothing they've done that you can't. In these pages I will offer the very same type of training program that has not only worked for Demi Moore, but for many other of America's most visible and sought-after women.

I've designed specific post-pregnancy programs for actress Tatum O'Neal, noted TV journalist Maria Shriver (Mrs. Arnold Schwarzenegger) as well as Patti Scialfa (the wife of Bruce Springsteen). To completely enhance and sculpt their bodies, I've devised personal workouts for comedian Whoopi Goldberg, singer Belinda Carlisle, as well as super-model Christy Turlington.

Exactly When Should You Start

One of the first questions I usually get from my clients is when should they begin the post-pregnancy training program. Would it be best to start a few days after giving birth? A few weeks? Or should they wait at least several months? The first thing I tell them is to consult their physician to make certain. If you're in reasonably good health, there's no reason why you can't begin working out fairly soon after having a child. But let me strongly emphasize that if you've had a cesarean section and wish to start this workout within a few weeks of giving birth, make sure to get the approval of your doctor first.

I've had clients come to me many months—or even years—after giving birth, feeling a little guilty that it's taken them so long to begin an exercise routine. If you fall into this category, first get rid of that guilt. It's never too late to start. In fact, I've placed women on the post-pregnancy training program long after having a child, and guess what? They look and feel better than ever!

So isn't it time to say good-bye to that bulging belly forever? Isn't it time to start feeling more energized and less fatigued? Isn't it time to pack up those maternity clothes once and for all? But most important, isn't it time to start taking better care of yourself so that you can stay healthy and fit for the rest of your life?

I'm proud to say that my wife, Debra, will be featured as the sole model for this book. And I think you'll agree with me that she looks sensational for a woman who's had three children. However, not only has she maintained and even accentuated her appearance, through training Debra has increased her stamina and lowered her stress level as well. And because of this, she can give so much more to our children and me. The bottom line is that the post-pregnancy training is not only a special gift to yourself, it's a special gift of love and caring to those dearest to you.

> If you had a normal delivery, you can begin the post-pregnancy training about two weeks after giving birth. However, if there were complications, such as a cesarean, then you will have to wait about six to eight weeks before you can start. In any event, don't start my program before first determining your present level of fitness, preferably with a medical exam.

You Can't Trade in Your Body

Stars have a solid investment in their bodies. And you should feel exactly the same way. Think of your body as an expensive vehicle that you rely on every day. Without the proper preventive maintenance, it will eventually break down. Small things such as changing the oil, having regular tune-ups, even washing and waxing can all make a critical difference in how your car performs. Which is why, if you try to shortchange your body, it'll cost a lot more to fix than a Chevy.

I never accept the excuse that there's no time for working out. There's time, all right, but it has to be the right workout.

I've tailored this unique program to meet your specific needs at this very special moment in your life; a program you can start slowly and gradually increase at your own speed. You are going to have thoroughly invigorating workouts, unique exercises practically every single day which are going to stimulate dynamic new growth in your muscles. Even more inspiring, you will never duplicate the same routines two days in a row, since I've also made it a priority to eliminate the boredom that accompanies so many other types of training programs.

Since weight training is one-dimensional and lacks stimulation, you won't find me at the gym every day pumping iron. It's been my experience that mind-numbing, repetitive regimens are the number-one reason people drop out of an exercise program. Consequently, I've devised a totally specialized approach, incorporating an ever-changing and challenging menu of both indoor and outdoor activities. A simple system that allows all kinds of women to design a personalized workout all their own.

Not one part of you will be overlooked. I will provide a wide array of body-sculpting exercises for toning the stomach as well as contouring the thighs and buttocks after giving birth. I will show how to marvelously build up all your chest, arms, and leg muscles. What's more, I will detail fabulous methods guaranteed to fortify your poise, posture, and overall appearance through strengthening the neck, shoulders, and lower back. But this is only half the story. Supporting these refinements on the outside will be some remarkable advances on the inside.

Significant improvements in the cardiovascular, respiratory, and circulatory systems, a lower percentage of body fat, plus a better quality of life measure the true success of a fitness program. It's ultimately these profound changes, not only the slimmed-down thighs or the tightened buttocks, that help motivate individuals toward making a daily commitment to their health and well-being for the rest of their lives.

But Let's Get Beyond the Physical

However, an exercise program must not only be powerful in the physical sense; it must be *empowering* at the same time. From firsthand experience with many of the world's most photographed women, I have learned that simply looking terrific means remarkably little unless its accompanied by a clear sense of purpose, an inner vision that extends well beyond the physical.

After giving birth, you'll discover that sustaining a vigorous and challenging exercise program brings many rewards and breakthroughs. It produces invaluable habits such as self-discipline, plus a determined mind-set which can help surmount adversity, defeat, and disappointment.

From my fourteen years as a personal trainer, I've discovered that confidence and a strong sense of self-esteem flow from within, not without. A perfect body should only be a true reflection of the assurance inside, not a convenient way to mask nagging insecurities and doubts.

Of course, the improvements in your appearance that occur during the post-pregnancy training are splendid motivational tools. When people begin to look and feel better, they immediately achieve a whole new level of acceptance. They feel less self-conscious. Consequently they take more risks and worry less about rejection. While many of my clients focus on the weight they've lost after having a child, or higher muscle definition, to me the most important changes are still the ones that occur inside their heads—the positive mental attitude.

Without a doubt, the goals realized during this training will assist you enormously in preparing for whatever other goals you desire throughout your life.

The Choice Is Yours

Now it's time for you to make a choice. The first step is always the hardest, but if you decide to get with the program, I can absolutely assure you that the body you've always envisioned will become less of a dream and more of a reality. It's the same guarantee I gave Demi. It's the same guarantee I gave Madonna. It's the same guarantee I give all my clients. And it's the same guarantee I give to you. Because from this day forward, consider yourself one of my clients.

In the following pages, I will personally guide you through the same training methods that have so dramatically helped all my clients after their deliveries. But don't worry. There's nothing complex or mysterious to learn. Although my program is systematic, it's even easier than you would imagine. In fact, it's downright fun—a great way to achieve all the results you have every right to expect, and one that you can stick with for life.

From the first stretch through the final exercises, I'm sure you'll find my approach all-inclusive and enjoyable. I'm one hundred percent committed to giving even the most sedentary people everything they need to obtain the results they've always wanted, but until now thought were out of reach.

In short, you don't have to be a superstar to take full advantage of my post-pregnancy training program, but there's one thing that's absolutely certain—you sure will feel like a *superstar* if you do!

> **Remember, it's never too late to get into great shape, whether it's five days after giving birth—or five years!**

CHAPTER 1

Training in the Spotlight

It all started with Madonna. She recruited me in 1987 just before her much anticipated and publicized "Blond Ambition" tour. Until that time she had been doing a fitness routine consisting mostly of some jogging and aerobic classes, but these really didn't satisfy her ultimate goals or needs. The problem was that she just wasn't challenging herself to the fullest. After her first major series of stage outings she came to appreciate how vital health and fitness were to the success of her performances. Consequently with Madonna, as with all my clients, it was important to focus on stamina, endurance, and overall body shape as primary objectives.

When I first began training Madonna she was beautiful. She had the curves of a voluptuous Marilyn Monroe type, and this was her Hollywood-inspired image when she first burst upon the scene. However, Madonna wanted to change that. She wanted a leaner, stronger look.

Madonna wanted sleek muscularity but not greater mass. Therefore, I devised a cross-training schedule that alternated running, cycling, and weight-lifting, plus a host of flexibility exercises.

By the time she premiered on Broadway, starring in the hit play *Speed the Plow,* Madonna had slimmed down and replaced her soft curves with lean, well-distributed muscle. One clear example was her midsection. Here she had worked vigorously to develop a lovely V, that distinctive shape stomach muscles take when they're in perfect condition. All in all, Madonna was in fabulous form!

Demi: Less Is Moore

Demi Moore first contacted me in 1990 while I was still on the road with Madonna. At the time Madonna was probably the most photographed woman in the world, and Demi had heard about the trainer she was working with. But as it turned out, both of our schedules were so hectic at the time that I didn't actually have a chance to meet Demi until 1991, while she was already pregnant with her second child. Demi was scheduled to star in *A Few Good Men* two months after she gave birth, and she wanted to make certain she could be ready for the film when it began shooting.

From the very first minute we met there was an instant rapport between us. At twenty-eight years of age, Demi's immediate goal was to have a stronger and leaner image. Furthermore, she realized how crucial it was to bounce back right after giving birth.

Also during this period I started developing a good relationship with Bruce Willis, who is married to Demi. In fact, Bruce was so impressed with the results of his wife's training that he hired me to get him into top physical shape as well. I worked with him throughout the filming of such movies as *Die Hard* and *Pulp Fiction*. However, since Bruce has never been pregnant, I'll get back to Demi.

> Demi's *Vanity Fair* cover was a great statement for women. Just because you're pregnant doesn't mean you're not sexy. It was a bold, glorious photograph, taken seven months into Demi's second pregnancy. It shattered old myths and established a major milestone at the same time.

Converting Baby Fat to Fabulous Muscle

After her daughter's birth, I put Demi on an individualized training program. First on my list was building stamina, so I started her running for twenty minutes each day, which I gradually brought up to an hour. To keep her legs in great shape, I had her switch running techniques, performing intervals (sprinting that is alternated with easy jogging) as well as running up and down hills. For working the gluteal muscles, in addition to those of the inner and outer thigh, I had her side-stepping as well. (Don't worry. I'll explain all of this a bit later on.)

During Demi's training, I also concentrated on more exacting muscle definition, especially in the stomach area. On separate days we'd focus on the upper abs, lower abs, and the obliques, and on the fourth day we'd work the entire abdominal region.

There's no doubt the effort paid off. She bounced back into shape leaner and more muscular than ever before, yet absolutely voluptuous. As a matter of fact, months after she gave birth to her second child, Demi had the self-confidence (not to mention the outstanding figure) to pose for the cover of *Vanity Fair* wearing nothing but a painted-on suit. If you saw that picture, you can judge for yourself how successful we were at whittling away all that baby fat—even after two pregnancies.

Working out not only keeps Demi in beautiful shape, but also aids in keeping her alert and mentally focused—qualities that are pivotal for success in the movie business, and any other business, for that matter. This is why the post-pregnancy training is absolutely vital for the woman who wants to pursue a professional career as well as motherhood. The workout produces not only great physical shape but keeps your mind fit as well. Since your ability to concentrate is enhanced, every aspect of your life is improved.

I believe one of the major reasons for the success of my program is the wide range of choices I offer my clients. For example, I expanded Demi's training to include kayaking and waterskiing, two summer activities that she already enjoyed to begin with. When winter came along, I had her take up skate-skiing and snow-shoeing—two very strenuous endeavors. Beating the drudgery of exercise is what my training is all about. I don't enjoy being in a gym all day long, nor do my clients, and neither does Demi.

Of course, like many other people, Demi can sometimes overly focus on her weight. That's why I stress during our training sessions that weight by itself is not the issue; it's how the weight is distributed, what percentage is fat, and what percentage is muscle. So my approach centers much more on shaping and toning than on losing weight just for the sake of losing weight.

Putting Your Priorities in Order

I've seen Demi through a number of great films, including *Indecent Proposal, A Few Good Men, Disclosure, The Scarlet Letter,* and *The Juror.* In my opinion her physical condition only keeps getting better and better because she's made working out regularly a top priority in her life. If Demi has to be on the set at 6:00 A.M., we'll train at 4:00 A.M.; if she had to be on location at 4:00 A.M., then we'd start at 2:00 A.M. No matter what her schedule, Demi fits training into it.

Now, I know some of you may be thinking, "Of course she can fit exercise in; she probably has a whole staff of hired help to take care of her children." Not true! During the time I trained Demi, I discovered that our outlooks on parenting are remarkably similar. I think we both believe in the singular importance of spending quality time with your children—of making them the number one priority in your life.

Even with all her traveling, Demi made sure that there was never a major separation away from her family. Both Demi and Bruce are incredibly devoted parents who agree that it's just not worth it to be apart from their kids for a prolonged period of time. They put their kids to sleep at night and get them up in the morning, just like any other loving parents would do.

As you can see, despite her status as an international star, Demi is really very down-to-earth. There's no one who's going to take care of her baby except her and Bruce. There's no twenty-four-hour child care assistant at their house; they're the ones up in the middle of the night whenever one of their children is crying or needs a glass of water.

In terms of scheduling her workouts, Demi has had to balance her time between her baby girls and training just like any other busy mother would. One thing that makes it easier is that Demi simply views exercise as a part of her life—just like having lunch or taking a shower. Sometimes she works out while the babies are napping. Other times Demi exercises before they wake up in the morning or after they go to sleep at night. Also, she and Bruce take turns watching the kids while the other spends an hour or two training. The bottom line is that when working out becomes as natural and necessary as, say, brushing your teeth, you don't have to make a choice, you just have to make the time.

> **The primary reason Demi trains is not for vanity's sake, but because she really knows how much her health and well-being will ultimately benefit her family.**

Oh, That Tatum O'Neal

One evening Madonna was having dinner with Tatum O'Neal and John McEnroe. The subject turned to physical fitness and my name came up. Tatum had given birth to two children, and now she wanted to get her pre-pregnancy body back. Madonna highly recommended me, and several months later Tatum and I were working together.

Tatum had always been a natural athlete. Raised as a tomboy, she could shoot up a flight of stairs, dash across a running track—you name it. But like other folks who spend time raising children, she had allowed herself to get a little out of shape. Although she was somewhat soft in spots, Tatum was determined to get back to where she was, and this time stay there.

The training we did closely resembled the workout I did with Demi, and soon the dramatic improvement began to show. Tatum dropped several dress sizes while she firmed up her thighs, arms, and waistline. Her stamina increased remarkably, and she literally had tons of newfound energy. The change was so profound even her husband was impressed. And so then John McEnroe asked me to train him as well.

I remember one magazine photo from a few years ago. Tatum (looking just fantastic) is immersed in a swimming pool with a lifesaver around her neck. And when you read the caption, it quotes her as saying that I was a "lifesaver" to her. Well, it's small things like that that make my job an absolute joy!

Patti Scialfa: Trained in the USA

I believe Patti found out about me through an article in *People* magazine. After our first meeting she decided to hire me—probably because I didn't come across like a drill sergeant. Since I've worked with so many clients during their post-pregnancy periods, I have a unique understanding of what they're experiencing at this time, both emotionally and physically, so this contributed to our initial rapport.

Both during and after her pregnancy Patti's energy was low and she was experiencing lower back problems, weakness, and pain, which is not at all unusual. As a result of her recurrent difficulties, she had stopped jogging. Patti thought she would never be able to get back into a running program, which was a shame because this was something she had once really enjoyed. So with Patti, the work was really cut out for me.

The first thing I did was address her lower back concerns by establishing a routine of abdominal work. Often by simply strengthening this specific area, much of the strain on the back muscles can be alleviated, resulting in far less discomfort. In order to improve her flexibility, we started working in the pool a lot. Then for stamina we began taking hikes, which I made progressively more challenging. When combined with the abdominal training, this specialized workout program considerably alleviated Patti's lower back distress. Her back felt better than it had for a long time.

Soon we started implementing a running program. And the great thing was her back didn't give her any problems. By sticking to our original training schedule she had built a good foundation, which now enables her to jog six or seven miles at a session.

I think Patti is an inspiring example of someone who surmounted a chronic problem through exercise. Whether it's lower back pain or fatigue, headaches or insomnia, this training program can remedy many of your most annoying conditions.

> **Remember: The investment that you make in yourself through training pays back a hundredfold.**

Maria Shriver

Maria and I have worked together for more than eight years, and she is quite an extraordinary woman. She originally came to me through Tatum. Maria saw the progress Tatum had made after giving birth and decided she wanted to expand her exercise program.

Since I have known her, Maria has had three children—in fact, she had three children over a period of three and a half years. This made her training program quite unique. We had to continually adjust her exercise regimen; the workouts evolved as she went from pre-pregnancy, through the different stages of pregnancy, to post-pregnancy. After giving birth to her first child, we had a short period where we worked out intensely. When she became pregnant the second time, we had to slow down the pace without giving up efficiency. By the time she became pregnant with her third child, we knew exactly what to do to maintain her level of fitness. But whether we were working hard or at a more moderate level, Maria made sure that she was always doing something— even if it was just walking.

I see Maria practically every day—usually the first thing in the morning. Maria's goal is to increase her overall fitness and maximize her stamina. She is no different than any other woman in that she has to meet the demands of juggling work, marriage and children. With her challenging career, three young children, and an equally active and successful husband, it is important that she maintain her energy level. To do this, we do a combination of hiking, biking and strength training. Just as important, this program helps Maria feel good about herself and her body.

Maria is seriously involved with a number of organizations that promote healthy lifestyles for both children and adults. On a more personal level, she strongly believes in giving the gift of fitness as well. Through the years I've been very gratified by the fact that Maria has given many of her friends—as a present—personal training sessions with me. I'm deeply honored by her continued faith and support all these years.

"If I Were Rich, I Could Have a Personal Trainer, Too"

Of course you could. But no matter what you believe about fame and fortune, all my clients have simply made the decision to put fitness at the top of their list. Listen, I'm not doing it for them. *They* are doing it for themselves. And in the following pages I will show you exactly how to do the same thing for yourself. In the end, money has very little to do with it. But the willingness to finally take charge of your health and well-being certainly does.

CHAPTER 2

No More Exercises
in Futility

I doubt if there's an excuse that I haven't heard about why women don't exercise after giving birth, or why they stop training only a few months after they start. Working out is an activity, but there are many women out there who have adopted a secret philosophy of passivity. This doesn't mean they let others push them around or that they can't defend themselves. It doesn't even imply that they aren't ambitious. Being passive means that you offer excuses for not taking complete charge of your health and well-being. And from what I've seen, these are often very rational, very-well-thought-out excuses. Too bad I don't buy any of them.

If you're looking for a trainer who's sympathetic to the fact that your newborn baby or children take up all your time, that you work twelve hours a day, or that you're out of town twice a month, then you'll have to look somewhere else. I don't coddle my clients. I don't care how rich or famous or busy they are.

> When I take on a client, it comes not only with a commitment to me, but with a commitment to themselves. And believe me, I never let them back out without a fight!

And don't think I'm going to treat you any differently. I know you can do it. I've headed up the sports training division of one of the country's most prestigious health facilities. I've seen thousands of my students come and go. They've come in overweight and out-of-shape, lacking in energy and motivation, and left looking years younger with a renewed sense of vitality. I've personally worked with women who are stockbrokers, lawyers, teachers, doctors, and top fashion models, all of whom had killer schedules plus a family to raise.

Certainly I've trained extremely successful and motivated people, but I've also devised programs for women who have abused drugs and alcohol, who were miserably depressed or consumed by anxiety after their pregnancies. Day after day, week after week, I've witnessed how they've turned their lives around, creating a positive sense of self and a reason to strive forward.

So right off the bat, don't tell me you can't do it. **You can do it.** And I will be here every step of the way to make sure you do. At first you'll hear my voice telling you to push yourself more and more, to break through those self-imposed walls and mental blocks. But pretty soon it will be your own voice you hear. A confidant, in-charge voice that will resonate within your head and literally become part of your life.

> **Always recognize that there are never any limits to what you can accomplish, only the limits you place upon yourself.**

Expanding the Exercise Menu

Maybe you're not quite sold yet. I don't blame you. It took years to build up those walls, those excuses for failing at an exercise program, and they're not going to tumble down overnight. But what we can do is start removing one brick at a time so that you can get a clear view of what's on the other side.

The main reason clients of mine have stopped previous workout programs has been out of sheer boredom. One leading film executive I train spent over two thousand dollars on her computerized exercise bicycle. It had all the bells and whistles, a heart-rate and blood-pressure monitor, plus a virtual reality program that created a fantasy bike race which allowed her to compete practically anyplace in the world. Needless to say, the bike has been collecting dust in her closet for the past two years. Another client of mine, a prominent Beverly Hills psychologist, invested in an expensive treadmill for herself and, sure enough, quickly ran out of patience.

Equally disastrous results await those who buy rowing machines or who expect to faithfully follow aerobic or step programs on celebrity videotapes. The boredom factor comes into play very quickly. You just can't do the same workout over and over and over again. Even the most committed joggers I know often have to fight off a sense of tedium, as if they were running around in circles.

> Is it any wonder many of us share W. C. Fields's wry observation, "Every time I get the urge to exercise, I lie down and wait till it passes."

Variety is not only the spice of life, but the major ingredient in a productive training program—which is good news. It means that you can finally drag your rowing machine or stair climber out of the garage and incorporate it into your workout, but in a fresh and dynamic way.

I believe each day of exercising should be a unique challenge. You wouldn't eat the same meal every night. So why should your menu of exercise only serve up one dish? As we carefully design your individual program, I will show you how to cook up a gourmet platter of post-pregnancy workouts that will keep you involved year in and year out, for the rest of your life.

Getting Those Walls to Tumble Down

Like many of my clients who recently gave birth, you may fall into the category of those people who got off to a terrific start, only to be sidetracked by a hectic work schedule or personal crisis. You were just going great, but then your routine was disrupted and somehow you've never gotten back on track. Perhaps your desire dies as you approach your goal. Before I started working with her, a very prominent screenwriter had a twenty-year pattern of first losing fifteen pounds and then putting them on all over again—and this happened at least three times a year.

I wish I could say hers was a unique case, but it's not. I see these self-defeating patterns over and over. Often women are not motivated by what's right with them, but what's wrong with them. They see their physical imperfections and needlessly dwell on them. Janice, an overseas sales rep for a large production company, was determined to start an exercise program after having a baby girl, but only after she dropped ten pounds. She said that she didn't want to appear to chunky at the gym, since she felt uptight around all the other women there.

Janice went on a liquid protein diet. But that eventually left her so weak that she passed out in a meeting with executives from a Japanese investment firm. After crunching her forehead on a mahogany conference table, and winding up in the emergency room needing twelve stitches, Janice finally saw the light. She decided to embark on a realistic course of physical fitness, without letting her embarrassment stifle her intentions.

When I first started with Janice, she still saw working out as compensation for her "imperfections." I immediately informed her this was a mistaken attitude. There was absolutely nothing wrong with her body. Her body wasn't bad, it wasn't her enemy. It was her colleague, her friend, her companion for life. I told Janice that she and her body should form a mutually supportive relationship. They should be buddies! Working together until their goals are realized. And from the start, I tell each of my clients exactly the same thing.

Unless there's some overriding genetic factors that make it impossible for you to change, unless you've been disabled in an accident or suffer from some grave illness, there's virtually no reason why you can't live up to your body's fullest potential. You aren't at war with your body after having a child—you are in partnership with it. Motivate yourself to stop playing the victim and start becoming the victor.

I don't blame anyone for not being in shape. One of the major factors causing weight gain is not just your pregnancy, but the aging process itself. You naturally accumulate a little more fat tissue with each year that passes. But this can be managed very easily. Fat can be zapped—it's as simple as that.

Don't Be a "Block" Head

We throw up all sorts of mental blocks along the way to optimum fitness. Is there anyone reading this who would deny that health is your most valuable possession? You can replace your condo, your Mercedes, even your poodle, but it's difficult to get your health back.

Every single workout involves a choice: either you're going to do it or you won't. You can always rationalize skipping a session or two for perfectly legitimate reasons: You need to get the baby some diapers. Your parents are in town. The latest episode of *Seinfeld* is on, or maybe the laundry is about to mildew. There are literally hundreds of ways you can talk yourself out of exercising after pregnancy. And each one sounds sensible and logical.

But add them up and you'll discover that you're severely short-changing yourself. I call every rational excuse you come up with for not exercising a *mental detour*. They can appear at any time—at the beginning of your journey, halfway there, or just when you're reaching your destination. There are no road signs along the way announcing mental detours, only feelings of inner dissatisfaction.

Surmounting mental detours requires reprograming the manner in which you view exercise and fitness. By identifying the patterns that control your basic attitudes, you can begin to reshape the course of your thinking. See if the following statements sound familiar.

Detours Along the Road to Fitness

- I admit it. I only work out seriously just before swimsuit season comes around.
- Of course I'd love to exercise all the time, but since my pregnancy, I'm afraid that my responsibilities are simply not compatible with a regular workout routine.
- I don't care what anyone says, exercise is plain boring. I go crazy from all the repetition. My idea of hell is to be stuck on a rowing machine for thirty minutes.
- All right, all right, I know training is important. But my parents simply didn't teach me self-discipline or willpower.
- If you ask me, I think exercise is great. It's the most important thing you can do. Too bad it seriously cuts into the quality time I spend with my newborn.

- Aerobics, are you kidding? Have you seen what my butt looks like in a leotard!
- Sure, I could look like Cindy Crawford, but it's such an effort!

Exertion Plus Exercise Equals Ecstasy

One of the first mental blocks that interfere with this special workout program is the fear that exercise is strenuous. Of course it's strenuous—but the more strenuous, the more joyous. Now, I'm not implying you immediately have to challenge a mountain or go white-water rafting through the Grand Canyon. Each one of us has a barrier to move through, and as we do, we gather momentum to go through the next one and then the next.

The first step is to set a realistic goal for yourself. Maybe it's doing ten sit-ups by the end of a week, perhaps five sets of forearm curls with three-pound weights. It doesn't make a difference. With every goal reached there comes a new confidence and spirit of achievement. Together with fat and cellulite, you can vanquish old fears and anxieties.

Nevertheless, as others react favorably to the changes they see, there is always the danger of focusing exclusively on your outward appearance. Indeed, the majority of Americans view "looking good" as the single most important benefit of an exercise program. However, it's actually the *least* important. I'll say that again. Becoming more physically attractive and desirable should be way down on your list of priorities, because there are far more lasting and significant reasons to be fit.

They fall into four basic categories. Repeat each one to yourself. Memorize them if you can. Make them part of your belief system, and remember: What you want is ultimately what you'll get.

Consistently set reasonable goals for yourself and you won't be disappointed. Losing about a pound a week is a reasonable goal; dropping down four dress sizes by the end of the month is not.

1. Optimum Physical Gains

- I want to experience boundless energy, a new threshold of stamina and vitality that I've never felt before.
- I want to expand dynamically the sheer power of my muscles, improve my endurance, and increase my athletic capacity.
- I want to develop my sense of coordination, and in the process I want all my reflexes to be more alert, my responses sharper to anything that might come my way.
- I want my body to move with grace and style, balance and poise, a strong sense of bearing and self-confidence.
- I want to reduce or eliminate the misery of low back pain, as well as get rid of other body aches and annoyances.

2. Optimum Health Gains

- I want to slash the percentage of fat in my body, and be certain that I'm never overweight again. I want to stop yo-yo dieting, which is dangerous to my health.
- I want to lessen my chances of developing heart problems, dramatically lower my overall blood pressure, strengthen my cardiovascular system, and make sure that the circulation to each of my organs is maximized to the fullest.
- I want to stop tossing and turning at night and sleep more restfully, ready to face each and every morning with renewed strength and vigor.
- I want to stop getting sick so often, and fortify my immune system against disease and infection.
- I want to release feelings of stress, stop being so nervous, and alleviate headaches and tension in my body.

3. Optimum Mental Gains

- I want to achieve much more without becoming exhausted, and have the ability to counter feelings of weariness and fatigue.
- I want to beef up my confidence for physical challenges such as tennis, racquetball, golf, hiking, and skiing.

- I want to magnify my intellectual agility, and be able to focus with greater amounts of clarity.
- I want to boost my self-esteem to record levels, and feel completely sure of myself, no matter what the situation.
- I want to experience the feeling of being totally in control of my life, the invigoration of really knowing that I'm taking total responsibility for my health and well-being.

4. Optimum Economic Gains

- I want to minimize the amount I spend on medical concerns, including doctors' bills and prescriptions.
- I want the lowest rates on the premiums I have to shell out for health insurance.
- I want to increase my overall productivity through decreasing the time I'm out sick and under the weather.
- I want to raise my powers of concentration so that I can better focus on making the right career and investment choices for myself.

Motivation vs. Willpower

Right now you're probably exhausted most of the time. Small wonder achieving goals after having a child is more difficult than setting them. Laying out the course is easy, but crossing the finish line is another matter. I've found there's a general misconception that equates motivation with willpower, and sometimes it's this very confusion that defeats us even before we start.

By definition, willpower implies expending enormous amounts of energy just to get ourselves in motion. Put another way, willpower simply means self-discipline. And let's be honest, all of us simply despise any form of discipline.

But motivation is quite different. When you feel motivated there is a strong desire to excel and improve. Your efforts become clearly focused on finding out how to feel better, initiating action rather than torturing yourself by exerting loads of willpower.

Motivation is a process that requires effective thinking, an expanded state of mind directed specifically toward getting results. Men and women who think effectively don't pursue perfection, they seek excellence. In much the same way, if you only seek the perfect body, then you will never be satisfied. In fact, you will constantly torment yourself.

> **Don't expect to slim down to Claudia Schiffer's size within a couple of weeks or look like Cindy Crawford by bathing suit season. Those goals are not only unrealistic, they're self-defeating.**

Only Compete with Yourself

You're not exercising to look as good as your sister, your best friend, or even a TV or movie star. Your goals are unique and they apply only to you. It's not about competition—who can lose weight the fastest or have the flattest stomach—it's about individual performance and excellence. The willingness to fulfill your ultimate fitness potential. One person's goal might be to run the New York City marathon in less than four hours; another's could simply be walking up a flight of steps without huffing and puffing. Everyone's aims are different.

If the bottom line is making someone else's approval your major goal, then you'll quickly run out of steam. The passion will be lost and you'll wind up frustrated. First give yourself a level of difficulty you can handle. Don't worry about what anyone else thinks. Perhaps the greatest aspect of the post-pregnancy training program is that you're not performing for yourself. What you achieve is private and confidential—until you decide to let the world know.

I've had clients who have come to me completely distraught after taking an aerobics class. Here they were, ten, twenty, maybe even forty pounds overweight after having a child, and they were subjected to an environment in which they immediately felt inadequate. Some of them even left in tears.

Whenever I work with a client, we train in a safe space, where no one else can observe us. As you progress through this book, I recommend that you set up a safe space as well, a place where you feel secure and protected as you exercise. This will prevent curious eyes from distracting or judging you. Find a time that's best for you, one that best fits into your schedule; but once you make that plan, agree to stick to it.

If you decide waking up forty-five minutes early is the only way to get your routine in, then go to sleep forty-five minutes earlier. Should evenings work better, then by all means work out then. There's really no right or wrong, only what's right or wrong for you.

The Point of Commitment

Simply trying to be in shape doesn't work for very long. The word *trying* itself implies that you are imposing some outside form of behavior on your true nature. In short, you're forcing yourself. How many times have you "wanted" to go on a diet? How many times have you "promised" that you were going to get physically fit? You keep repeating that you desire change. But "desire" is not enough, either.

Beyond "trying," beyond "wanting," even beyond "promising" and "desiring," there is the point of commitment. Notice that *commitment* is not a verb, it's a noun. It's a state of mind, a description of consciousness, not an action or feeling. Commitment is not an effort. It's not a decision. It's a process by which you've decided to get where you're going, without being sidetracked by where you've been.

Commitment requires a compelling and inspiring purpose in order for you to be consistent in your training. This purpose must represent a powerful and constant reminder of the mighty benefits of being in great shape, a reason to overcome the temptation to slack off. All too often I find women have not entirely formulated a precise picture of their ultimate goals after their pregnancy.

Instead I often hear general statements such as "I want to take inches off my butt" or "I want to look sexy for my sister's wedding" or even "I want to get back to how I looked in college." Not that these aren't worthy goals. It's just unlikely that any of them, all by themselves, will sufficiently motivate you to pursue a program of lifelong fitness.

When starting the post-pregnancy training, try to see the big picture. What are your long-term goals? Is it really just losing ten pounds in a month? Are you actually preoccupied with fitting into a size six? Or is there something much greater at stake? Something so vital that any excuse for not working out seems almost trivial by comparison.

> One positive way of making a strong commitment to your post-pregnancy training schedule is by focusing on the eventual benefits, not the exercises themselves.

Lifting ten-pound weights may appear rather masochistic if you're not driven by a higher purpose. Jogging at six in the morning—when there's hardly another soul around—can also seem senseless. To clarify the reasons behind your commitment, check over the following list of questions.

Take a piece of paper and jot down the answers that most apply to your situation. I've discovered that putting down your long-range goals in black and white clarifies and strengthens your commitment to fitness, while identifying obstacles and barriers. After you finish, take a few minutes to look over your responses. See if there's any pattern you can identify. Is there a common thread that ties all of your answers together? If you're like most people, there definitely is a common denominator.

Finding Powerful Reasons for Commitment

1. In what ways would an exercise program have a positive effect on your family life? Your sex life? Your relationships with your spouse, children, parents, or other relatives?
2. How could working out benefit your productivity at work? How could it possibly help advance your career?
3. Do you want more respect and recognition from your friends? How would training help supply what's currently missing from your life?
4. Is there someone you want to particularly impress? Why is their approval so important?

5. Are you driven by a burning desire? An aspiration that eclipses everything else? In what way will working out facilitate this goal and make it a reality?

6. How would post-pregnancy training assist you in breaking through other blocks that stop you from performing at 100 percent? What are those blocks? Where do they come from? What would your life look like without them holding you back? What would be the ripple effect?

7. How would exercising expand your potential for living? What things would you attempt that you never tried before? Where would you go that you've never been before? Who would you be with that you've never been with before?

8. Were you once in terrific shape? Have you let yourself go? Would post-pregnancy training help you return to the shape you were in? Why is that significant? What would that prove?

9. How will working out persistently improve your self-esteem? How will it combat the fear that you're a loser? That you're a quitter? That you don't have what it takes to make it? How will training make you more resilient? More able to take a punch and then get back on your feet?

10. Is post-pregnancy training your ticket to long life? Can you see yourself remaining active and energetic well into your sixties? Your seventies? Your eighties? Are there specific health concerns that run in your family, such as obesity or high blood pressure? How will physical training lessen the chances of developing heart disease or other serious disorders? Will working out help you defeat other destructive behavior, for instance, drinking or using drugs?

How to Use Your Responses

Incorporate your responses into developing a personal strategy, the reasons behind your commitment. Once it becomes clear you can get past all the resolutions you've ever broken, all the false starts you've ever made. Making a commitment to fitness after giving birth doesn't mean a month, a year or even a decade. It's a lifelong process, one that doesn't mean eternal suffering, but tremendous exuberance every single day. Being committed truly extends beyond the negatives. It's the transition from "doing" to "being."

The Temptation to Slack Off

Nevertheless, even the strongest commitment can occasionally falter. I've had some clients who were under the impression that once they got into top shape they could take off for a little while without worrying too much. But I quickly informed them otherwise. It only takes a month after you stop working out to put your health in jeopardy. First of all, the muscles begin to atrophy, your energy drops substantially, not to mention your heart and lung capacity also begins to decline.

What's worse, you lose your motivation. You start becoming upset with yourself, a little more each day. As a matter of fact, you might even punish yourself until the body on the outside begins to reflect the state of mind inside. There's only one thing worse than not exercising at all, and that's starting a workout program but never completing it. You invariably wind up calling yourself a quitter. Your self-esteem suffers. And it becomes tougher and tougher to begin all over again.

What it all boils down to are your preconceptions. As long as you perceive that exercise is not really worth the effort, that the stress and strain outweigh the benefits, then you won't be committed to exercise. The inconvenience alone will be enough of an excuse to sabotage your post-pregnancy workout.

It happens all the time. People exhaust incredible amounts of energy contemplating whether or not the current conditions are "ripe" for exercise. For instance, your health club is usually only a twenty-minute drive from the office, but it's really pouring outside, so let's put the workout off until tomorrow. Here's another example. After working really hard for the past six months raising a child, you've treated yourself to a cruise, two fabulous weeks of rest and relaxation with your family. There's no doubt about it. You've earned the break, especially a break from exercise.

But these types of conclusions are completely arbitrary. Because it was raining outside, you might have just as easily rationalized going to the gym by simply saying it was the "perfect" day for a workout. Similarly, concerning the cruise, you could have made your voyage a golden opportunity to intensify and fortify your quest for fitness without outside interruption, in the ship's gym.

The secret is in knowing that your basic attitudes can be reshaped as effectively as your physical appearance. When this happens you are not only conditioning your body, but your mind. You are teaching yourself to act in a positive, life-affirming way, refusing to surrender to feelings of anxiety or doubt. Training your mind to stay with a commitment is very much like winning a debate, point and counterpoint, until you literally talk yourself out of any self-defeating behavior. The following is an example:

Fighting Fire	*With Fire*
1. With all the diapers and the crying and the feedings, there's no use starting one now. I'll just wait until the baby gets older.	1. That doesn't make lots of sense. The longer I wait, the more out-of-shape I'll be. Then I'll have to work even harder.
2. This baby has left me totally exhausted. I can barely drag myself around, let alone start an exercise program.	2. Of course I'm exhausted. Have I ever considered the fact that exercising will give me tons of vitality?
3. Right now I'm on a diet. And whatever weight I can't lose, I'll simply have them nip and tuck or remove with liposuction.	3. I know diets are ineffective unless they're combined with regular exercise. And without working out, the cellulite will come back with a vengeance.
4. I admit it. I'm hopeless. I'm lazy, a real couch potato, and there's no power on earth that can budge me.	4. Oh, yes there is. All I have to do is imagine the life of an ultimate couch potato, strapped to a heart monitor in a hospital bed.
5. I haven't gone to the gym for two weeks. Something always seems to come up. I guess when it comes to working out, I'm a real loser.	5. Since when does my future progress have to be tied to my past performance? So I screwed up a couple of times. Big deal. Tomorrow I'm in the gym!
6. It's not fair. I'll never be a perfect 10, so why kid myself. No matter how many hours I spend in the gym, it just won't happen. So why even bother?	6. Very few individuals are perfect 10s. If I'm basing my self-esteem entirely on my looks, then shame on me. I've got a lot more to offer, so I better get my act together right away.
7. I'm really feeling too down today to work out. I'm feeling a little blue and out of it. I think I'll put off my workout for today.	7. I'm the mistress of my emotions, and they aren't going to prevent me from doing what I absolutely know is in my best interest! Plus those endorphins generated by training will really help brighten up my spirits!
8. My husband and kids are moaning and groaning that I'm not spending enough time with them. I'm really feeling guilty. Maybe I'm being selfish with this exercise program. I mean, I should be a wife and mother first, and Jane Fonda second.	8. I think it's time to call a family peace conference. First I will clearly explain why working out is absolutely vital and necessary. And second, I will organize a schedule that we all agree to, in order to share time together without sacrificing my goals.

Fighting Fire	*With Fire*
9. I accept that I'm a total screw-up. I've been that way since day one. I never really have any enthusiasm. Let's face facts. I've just got no willpower.	9. Maybe I've been a screw-up, but no more, my friend. I'm sticking to my training program. I'm going to prove that I can complete any project I choose. I can really enjoy life, if I just give myself half a chance.
10. Look at these hips. And my stomach hanging over my waist. Is it any wonder why I'm a social outcast? Why I'm so embarrassed all the time?	10. I could lose thirty pounds and what would be my excuses then? Look, I'm tired of staying home alone. I deserve to be with people. My goal is never to feel uptight around anybody ever again.
11. All the health clubs in my neighborhood are too expensive to join. They want initiation fees, and monthly deductions from my credit card. I'm not sure I can afford it.	11. Listen, I can't afford *not* to exercise. What's the cost to my health if I don't take charge of my body now. And who says I have to join a health club? There are all sorts of exercises I can do without even setting foot in a gym.
12. I'm a free spirit. I like to be totally spontaneous. Planning a training schedule is such a drag. It really cramps my style. I like to make last-minute decisions, you know what I mean?	12. I know what I mean. I'm really shortsighted. How long do I think I can enjoy my freedom? Come on. Get real. I better start training today so that my body doesn't really cramp my style!
13. I've got to admit it. I look pretty damn good. I've got no physical complaints. My body practically runs itself. Why do I need the headache of exercising?	13. Sure, I look good now, but the outside isn't everything. What about the inside? What's going on there? I better start training now so I can stay gorgeous for a long time to come.
14. Call it neurotic behavior. I'll start a project with a lot of positive energy, but all of a sudden my enthusiasm peters out. It's the same with exercise. I start off real strong, do everything at light speed, but then kind of lose steam and drop out.	14. Here's the decision I have to make. Am I really incapable of finishing anything? Do I have a fear of success? Is my true self a quitter? Well, there's one solid way to prove I'm not a loser. And that's by getting in shape, and staying in shape.
15. Exercise is so tedious, it's like anesthesia for my brain. I go numb. I can't do it. You would have to be a regular robot to get through all those exercises without keeling over. The boredom is excruciating!	15. There I go again. Making everything so dramatic. Instead I could be focusing on making my training a real blast, challenging and exciting. The truth is I'm responsible for my own experience. So get with the program. The only thing that's really boring is my attitude!

Putting It Down on Paper

The final step in becoming totally motivated is making a firm commitment to yourself. Unfortunately, these are the hardest agreements to keep. Signing a contract with a business partner or a lease with a landlord would literally impel you to live up to the conditions agreed upon. However, since a commitment is a contract with yourself, there's nobody around to enforce it. No one watching over your shoulder.

Until now, that is—because before embarking on this post-pregnancy fitness program, you are going to enter into a three-month agreement. And there's no negotiating the terms, either. It's an agreement to take charge of your life, recognize your potential, and take responsibility for realizing your dreams.

This is a contract between you and me. I expect you to sign it and date it. Keep the original for your records and then either mail or FAX a copy to me. I will countersign it, send it back to you, plus enclose a personal message of encouragement.

Through the following pages I will keep this commitment to you, if you keep this commitment to me. As we progress together, I will show you how to set realistic goals that can be precisely measured—from running a mile in ten minutes to swimming thirty minutes three times a week. I will explain how to increase those goals for speed and stamina, and then give you a simple way to chart your progress.

Accomplishing your aims inspires even greater feats of fitness, as you seek to surpass the results you've already achieved. Without goals, there is no measure of your advancement, no way of acknowledging the plateaus you've reached. Whether it's jogging or biking, the amount of weight you've lost or how many sit-ups you can perform, monitoring each of these areas stimulates your appetite for results. With your sense of commitment deepening every day, ambitions that once seemed far away will suddenly seem close and attainable.

In setting individual goals, everyone wants to know what the end result will be. Well, contrary to popular belief, there is no end result, no final achievement, no reaching the finish line. Your health and well-being simply don't have limits. Both are ongoing concerns for life—and that's a critical distinction to make. Because then you can't fail, you can't criticize yourself. By just deciding to make the effort, you have already succeeded, you have already met your goal.

So take the pressure off yourself. Love the changes as they happen. If you've set a goal of losing thirty pounds, then allow yourself to revel in every single ounce you drop. Be exuberant about the process; don't feel you have to whip yourself into shape after giving birth. It's not about pain, it's about pleasure, the joy of choosing a meaningful goal, finding a path to attain it, then relishing the knowledge you've acquired along the way.

By signing this contract, you've agreed to do away with all the false starts. You've agreed to break old habits, self-defeating routines, and neurotic excuses for yourself. You've further agreed that you've absolutely got what it takes. And finally, you've agreed that you're ready for an incredible breakthrough. All right. Talk is cheap. Let's get up to Parr!

Letter of Agreement

THIS AGREEMENT is made and entered into this _____ day of _____, by and between _____ (hereinafter called "The Trainee"), residing in _____ and Rob Parr (hereinafter called "The Trainer"), residing in Brentwood, California.

Witnesseth:

Whereas, THE TRAINER is a recognized authority in the field of health and physical fitness.

Whereas, THE TRAINEE seeks to become physically fit and healthy for the rest of her life after giving birth.

Whereas, THE TRAINER will detail a comprehensive program for achieving these stated goals of health and fitness.

Whereas, THE TRAINEE will follow THE TRAINER'S instructions to the best of her ability for a period of no less than ninety (90) days.

NOW, THEREFORE, in consideration of the premises, and for the mutual promises and covenants contained herein, the parties hereto agree as follows:

1. THE TRAINEE agrees to start the post-pregnancy training program within this book upon the date of signing this contract, not tomorrow, nor the day afterward.
2. THE TRAINEE agrees to make her best attempt to fully complete each of these exercises, not taking any shortcuts or making any excuses except for major emergencies.
3. THE TRAINEE agrees not to be intimidated by those who have been working out for a longer period of time.
4. THE TRAINEE agrees that making time for health and fitness is her number-one priority, not only for herself, but in consideration of those who love her.
5. THE TRAINEE agrees that the results far outweigh the difficulties and inconvenience of exercising.
6. THE TRAINEE agrees to completely motivate herself, and not just wait until the "mood" strikes her to work out.
7. THE TRAINEE agrees to practice and perfect the routines contained herein, and should frustrations arise, to work through them instead of abandoning the program.
8. THE TRAINEE agrees to put aside past failures and disappointments and focus on getting into shape here and now.

9. THE TRAINEE agrees to be solely responsible for her physical state of being, not blaming anyone else for her deficiencies, especially her parents, employers, spouse, or children.
10. THE TRAINEE agrees to set both short- and long-range goals, and to meet those goals by the time specified.
11. THE TRAINEE agrees to keep weekly records as performance levels progress and improve.
12. THE TRAINEE agrees to follow a nutritional plan that supports the above stated health and fitness goals.
13. THE TRAINEE agrees to create an overwhelming reason to exercise every time a temptation to skip exercise presents itself.
14. THE TRAINEE agrees that the pursuit of physical excellence directly contributes to achieving excellence in every other aspect of her life.
15. TERM OF AGREEMENT: The term of this agreement shall commence on the signing of this agreement and will continue for ninety (90) days. This agreement shall automatically renew for successive one (1) year periods upon the terms and conditions contained herein for life.
16. WARRANTIES AND REPRESENTATIONS: Both THE TRAINEE and THE TRAINER represent, warrant, and covenant that (i) they each have the full right and authority to enter into and fully perform this agreement in accordance with its terms; (ii) that both THE TRAINEE and THE TRAINER will not do anything which might limit, diminish, or impair the rights which either of them has acquired in this agreement.
17. ENTIRE AGREEMENT: This agreement constitutes the entire agreement of the parties pertaining to the subject matter herein contained and it supercedes all prior and contemporaneous, written or oral agreements, representations, and understandings between the parties.

MUTUALLY AGREED and entered into effective the _____ day of _____ by and between the parties whose signatures appear below.

_____
(Your Signature)

_____
Rob Parr

Mail to: Rob Parr
      253A 26th Street
      Suite 264
      Santa Monica, CA 90402

CHAPTER 3

Thick and Tired of It
(Or Everything You *Never* Wanted to Know About Fat)

Many women become victims of their excess poundage. They see it as some fundamental deficiency, a cellular flaw in their basic composition. The truth is that practically every human being on the planet has a strong, predetermined genetic tendency toward producing pound after pound of body fat (including all those actors and actresses you currently see running around on *Baywatch*).

This metabolic process dates back to the time of the cavemen—and of course the cavewomen. You see, without the body's ability to produce fat, our ancestors would have starved to death. Back then there were no McDonald's or Burger King drive-throughs scattered along every single freeway exit, nor were there refrigerators or a dozen other conveniences we routinely take for granted.

Most of our forebears' time was spent foraging for food, and often they went for long periods of time without any nourishment whatsoever. Body fat served a critical purpose as fuel. A thick layer of fat was also needed just for getting through the harsh winter months, not to mention an occasional Ice Age or two.

On top of that, since women were ultimately responsible for childbearing and making sure the race didn't die out, they were often fatter than men. Carrying the weight in the buttocks and the thighs helped insure that the fetus would be cushioned and protected and warm.

Obviously we've come a long way—but unfortunately our genes are still back in the Stone Age. The genetic messages we carry around today still reflect many of the conditions of thousands of years ago. Our fore-bears ate when they could, and their bodies were programmed to store fat in order to get them through long periods without food.

But for most of us these days, our next meal is often no farther than the distance between the couch and the refrigerator. And unfortunately, for millions of Americans, this seems to be the only exercise they get. Small wonder that as a nation we're constantly fighting the battle of the bulge.

Survival of the Fattest

How times have changed! Less than a couple of generations ago, about the time our grandparents came to this country, fat was in. Being over-weight meant you were wealthy, successful, a bona fide mover and shaker. Even more than good looks, being overweight was the number-one physical asset. Over the course of centuries, hefty females have con-tinually adorned the canvases of famous painters, hence immortalizing the image of the "Rubenesque" woman.

Food has been a scarce commodity throughout the centuries. Those who could lavish vast amounts of food on themselves were often en-vied—and emulated. People wanting to increase their social standing were obsessed with putting on pound after pound. Big bellies were flaunted. Boasted about. Jiggled with impunity at dinner parties.

Had television existed back then, we would have seen Donahue or Oprah featuring individuals trying to deal with the stigma of being slim, and all the prejudice that was directed against them. If you weren't fat, you weren't where it was at.

But fatness was far more than just a status symbol. Being over-weight was considered the very embodiment of good health. To sets of worried parents, doctors of the time prescribed overeating as the only sure way of curing children of disease. But their prescription was driv-en by fear. Over the course of history plagues have ravaged the globe, killing people by the hundreds of thousands. Victims would lose their appetite and gradually waste away. Consequently it was reasoned that if the body had ample layers of fat it could wait out the disease and pro-tect itself.

Now, these early physicians weren't entirely wrong. Fat is an emer-gency resource of energy. The typical male or female has a reserve supply of forty days of fat beneath their skin. Before central heating and electric blankets, this fat insulated the body from the ravages of winter. Plus it's gotten the human race through famines.

> Historians say that hunger probably brought more people to our shores than oppression. Is it any wonder our parents would tell us all the time, "Eat. Eat!" Most likely because they heard it from their parents.

Is Twiggy to Blame?

Back in the sixties a skinny little British model took the fashion world by storm, and almost overnight "thin was in." Whether her popularity was a reaction to more voluptuous movie stars of the fifties—such as Marilyn Monroe and Jayne Mansfield—I don't know. But I do know we're still feeling the fallout from those times.

Now I'm not blaming Twiggy herself, but ever since her appearance on the scene, weight has become a national obsession. Over the past thirty years people have become more conscious of their excess poundage than ever before. Which in some ways is good, but in other ways bad.

Eating disorders such as bulimia and anorexia have become much more common. Questionable diet fads have come and gone. Gut-busting gimmicks crop up almost every night on TV. And as a nation we've been conditioned to believe that pounds alone are the problem, but they're not.

Fat Is the Problem. Not Weight.

We've become slaves to the scales. We allow our weight to rule our behavior. This is ridiculous. The standard height and weight charts we've all been brought up with exert a curious type of tyranny over our lives. They tell you how many pounds you should weigh, but they don't tell you how many of those pounds should be fat.

Being overweight only refers to the difference between where you are and your ideal weight. But the really critical consideration is your percentage of body fat. During pregnancy your body naturally accumulated more fat. (Remember that cavewoman?) Now, in order to look and feel better, you need to replace that fat with lean muscle tissue.

Inch for inch, pound for pound, muscle tissue is actually far more compressed than fat tissue; it takes up less space. In other words, by replacing fat with muscle, you're actually making yourself much leaner and firmer, even though you may not be losing that much weight. This is crucial to realize. The scale is not your friend. As a sole measure of your fitness, the scale is useless and frustrating. It's more meaningful to notice how your clothes fit and how you feel. That's the real test of success.

I recall a former beauty queen turned real estate agent (I'll simply call her Janet) who came to me wanting to tighten her "fat stomach" after giving birth. She was perplexed because even though she weighed five pounds less than when she was in her twenties, she didn't look as attractive. In fact, it seemed her waist was larger and her bust was smaller.

Janet was 5 feet 6 inches and weighed 125 pounds, which, according to all the height and weight charts, was just perfect for her. The truth is Janet was not overweight; she was simply overly fat. Through careful measuring I was able to determine that 31 percent of her weight was in actuality fat, well above the recommended amount for women. The bottom line was that Janet didn't need to lose pounds, she needed to transform body fat into muscle. And with my training program, Janet did exactly that.

> Many Europeans are rather amused by the fanatical emphasis Americans place on weight, as if this was the sole defining characteristic of bodies. In countries like Sweden or Germany, greater concern is given to overall fitness; pounds are merely readings on a scale and relatively insignificant. Since there are myriad body types, compositions, and structures, Europeans contend that assessing yourself by "ideal" weight is both absurd and self-defeating.

I've Got You Under My Skin

So how do you know if you have a high percentage of body fat? The indications of being overly fat are all too common: protruding stomachs, handlebars over the hips, flabby arms and thighs, heavy ankles, etc. However, the most accurate (and unfortunately the most expensive) way of determining the percentage of body fat is through using the hydrostatic weighing process. For this procedure you are immersed in a large tub. Then afterward, through the use of elaborate equipment that measures such small items as residual lung volume of air, your body fat percentage is calculated.

Luckily, there is another procedure that can easily be performed by your doctor with fairly precise results. Using a device called a caliper, skinfold thickness is measured and this determines the amount of fat stored in the body. Common areas that are routinely evaluated include the center of the back (usually at the shoulder blades), the abdomen, as well as skin folds beneath the armpit, chest, and the rear of the upper arm. After this is done, the results are averaged according to a standard formula and your percentage of body weight that is fat is then determined.

Most experts agree that children under the age of twelve should not have body fat in excess of 12 percent of their weight. In adults the optimum amount of body fat for a man should be 15 percent or less, while women would do best striving for 19 percent or less. The major reason that women have 4 percent more is because of the fat they carry in their breasts.

Olympic athletes, ballet dancers, and marathon runners often have remarkably low amounts of body fat. Long-distance runners can weigh in with up to 8 percent body fat, and gymnasts can sometimes have a percentage as low as 1.5 percent.

But when does body fat really become excessive? Researchers have set standards here as well. A man with body fat in excess of 20 percent and women with more than 30 percent are classified as being overly fat, which leaves them ripe for some very unpleasant consequences including diabetes, heart disease, stroke, hypertension, arthritis, gallstones, as well as certain types of cancers.

Redistributing weight is more important than losing it. As you transform fat into lean muscle, you will literally be condensing yourself. Let's say you and your best friend both weigh 150 pounds, but you have more muscle tissue. Then you would definitely be wearing the smaller dress size. It's that simple.

Of course, the simplest and least expensive way of approximating whether or not you're overly fat is simply by pinching yourself. Wherever you suspect there's too much body fat, such as around the waist, the back of the arm, thigh or stomach, pinch the skin using your thumb and forefinger. Take a look and then make a visual estimate. If you're pinching more than an inch you're probably overly fat.

Fat Chance: It's All in the Genes

Well, I wouldn't be too quick to blame your ancestors for producing the cellulite on your thighs. There's no single omnipotent gene which is responsible for being overly fat. As of today, most medical research points to the fact that a complex number of factors lead to getting heavy—and all of these have to act in concert.

The really terrific news is that scientists have demonstrated that only thirty to forty percent of weight problems come from genetic factors, which means that sixty to seventy percent are manageable through changing your lifestyle. However, by changing your lifestyle, I don't mean just deciding to go on a diet. That could actually be the worst fitness decision you ever make.

The Diet vs. Exercise Controversy

Diets are great for losing weight—but not necessarily fat. Research has shown that dieting alone has a high inefficiency ratio of two to one. Stated another way, for every three pounds you lose, only one third will be fat. The rest is muscle, and this can be extremely hazardous to your appearance. For instance, take a well-known film personality I once trained. After giving birth, she had lost more than thirty pounds on a popular liquid protein diet. She had gotten down to her target weight but looked terrible. Her breasts, which only several months before had been firm and erect, were now sagging, and she had developed a pot belly to boot. Suffice it to say, there was only one person in town even more alarmed than she was—and that was her agent.

In the course of crash dieting she had lost some of the lean, muscular tissue that her body desperately needed to look healthy and attractive. The tissue that kept everything else in place. Like so many others she had become obsessed with her weight, to the detriment of her beauty. And even more ironically, she had actually increased her percentage of body fat while dropping pounds. But luckily the damage was reversible. After immediately putting her on a post-pregnancy training program, her muscle tissue was soon restored as well as some of the necessary weight.

The point is: Diets by themselves don't work. Only a diet combined with a finely tuned training program can demolish fat for the rest of your life. Therefore, the answer to those flabby bottoms remains the same. Keep those barbells and jogging shoes within reach.

Some Basic Thoughts on Nutrition

The elements of eating healthier and lighter are fairly well-known. Keeping your fat intake below 30 percent a day is absolutely essential. I would also suggest cutting down on red meats in favor of fish or poultry. Also, supplement your diet with a healthy dose of fruits, vegetables, fresh juices, and grains.

Finally, to absolutely guarantee that you are receiving all the nutrients you should, I recommend taking vitamin supplements and minerals. And remember to always check with your doctor before making any major dietary changes.

Winning at the Weight-Loss Game: Ten Rules

RULE #1: MOTHER DOESN'T ALWAYS KNOW BEST

Never put anything in your mouth if you're not already hungry. Your body is not a clock. It doesn't automatically have to be fed at certain times of the day, no matter what you've been taught. Only eat to the point of satisfaction, not fullness or discomfort, no matter who's encouraging you otherwise, including your mother.

RULE #2: DON'T GAIN WEIGHT BY STARVING YOURSELF

Sounds preposterous, but it's true. Your body is not as preoccupied with dropping ten pounds before your sister's wedding as it is with survival—pure and simple survival. Locked into your genetic makeup is a self-preservation program.

After only about twelve days on a crash diet, a red light goes off in your brain. Then what happens is your Basal Metabolic Rate (or BMR— the speed at which the body burns calories when it is resting) starts to decline. To make matters even worse, the body starts burning lean muscle mass as fuel in order to protect fat, because fat is seen as your primary source of long-term energy.

Which means if you decide to drastically decrease your calories (say by going on a liquid protein diet), your body will respond by lowering your BMR, sometimes by as much as 10 percent in a single day. All because it doesn't want you to starve to death. The bottom line is that, even as you diet, your basic capacity to lose weight could actually lessen. A frustrating prospect, to say the least.

RULE #3: YO-YO DIETING IS A NO-NO

Yo-yo dieting plays absolute havoc with your BMR, making weight harder and harder to lose each time you try to radically cut your calorie count. On extreme diets, which are interpreted as nothing less than a major famine by your entire nervous system, your body will try its utmost to conserve calories even to the point of depleting muscle mass. To respond to these crisis conditions, your BMR is then automatically lowered as you approach your target weight.

Now let's say you've made it; you've dropped those ten pounds in just two weeks and you return to your careful eating habits, making sure to know the precise amount of calories of everything that passes your lips. Well, guess what? Since your body has become so remarkably fuel-efficient, like a Cadillac that discovers it can function on the horsepower of a Honda Civic, it no longer needs the same amount of calories every day. It needs less. But unfortunately you don't eat any less. The bottom line is that your fat comes back even faster than before.

RULE #4: WHEN LOSING A POUND IS SOUND

I advise you to set a goal of losing no more than one pound a week. There is a general rule of thumb that determines how many calories a day you should have in order to accomplish this. A pound is equivalent to about 3500 calories. Consequently, losing a pound a week would mean consuming merely 500 calories a day less than normal. The numbers become even friendlier when factoring in exercise. Let's say you forsake one small portion of cherry pie (275 calories) and burn an additional 225 calories by easily jogging for twenty minutes. Add them together and there's your 500 calories, practically no sweat.

RULE #5: SLOW BUT STEADY WINS THE RACE

Slower weight loss is the best way to ensure long-lasting results and is the most healthy. There's a way to determine the maximum number of pounds you can safely shed each week. Weight loss that stands the best chance of being long-lasting occurs at the rate of 1 percent of body weight per week. Suppose you're a gal who weighs 130 pounds. Then the amount of weight you should lose each week shouldn't exceed 1.3 pounds.

RULE #6: SLIMMING DOWN YOUR EXPECTATIONS

Permanent weight loss, as opposed to crash diets, can sometimes seem agonizingly slow. There may be weeks when you don't lose an ounce, even though you've faithfully adhered to your diet and exercise schedule. Don't worry. This is all perfectly acceptable. If you get stalled for a week or two, it's only because your BMR is in a state of transition, not because you've failed in any way.

Should this happen just go off your diet for a few days, but eat sensibly. The worst thing you can do is starve yourself or try to survive on those liquid protein shakes. As I mentioned before, BMR responds to caloric intake. If you've been losing weight too rapidly, your BMR could be slowing down a bit, in which case you have to start eating a little more to eventually lose a lot more. Let a few weeks pass. Then go back to your original diet plan.

RULE #7: PASTA MAKES PERFECT

To help those fat molecules go up in flames, make sure to eat a diet that's loaded with carbohydrates such as pasta, fruits, and vegetables. Carbohydrates are then transformed into glycogen, a leading source of energy for your body. The more carbohydrates you consume, the more intensely you'll be able to perform the post-pregnancy training, and the more unwanted fat you'll zap.

RULE #8: YOU GOT TO HAVE TIMING

How many of us have skipped breakfast in the morning only to plop down in front of the TV later that evening with a heavy order of Shrimp Fried Rice and a couple of egg rolls? For decades nutritionists have informed us that eating heavily after 8:00 P.M. is a no-no. But of course try telling this to those who love to munch a bunch while staying up to watch Leno or Letterman. Even fans of Ted Koppel are not immune to late-night raids on yesterday's meat loaf.

Nevertheless, as they do in many parts of Europe and the Middle East, you should eat your largest meal at lunchtime and then your smallest at night, preferably a low-fat, high-carbohydrate meal, no fewer than three hours before bedtime.

Your basic metabolism reaches its lowest ebb during the evening and therefore has a harder time dealing with excess calories. Hence at night your body should be resting comfortably, not wrestling with a fruitcake at 3:00 A.M.

RULE #9: REPLACING BREAKFAST, LUNCH, AND DINNER

Our society has been programmed around three basic mealtimes. It's a convention we've all been raised with; yet who says that you have to be conventional? In the best of all possible worlds you would be able to avoid huge breakfasts, lunches, and dinners altogether and replace them with a series of smaller and more frequent meals during the day, sort of a series of healthy snacks.

This would keep your blood sugar stable and ensure that ravenous hunger doesn't periodically consume your thoughts. By consuming calories in miniature doses, your metabolism operates more efficiently and your energy doesn't falter, a big plus when working out.

RULE #10: THE DIETICIAN AS MAGICIAN

Not even your M.D. may know as much about weight loss as an R.D. (registered dietician). Now when I say registered dietician I don't mean one of those so-called "counselors" who inhabit assorted weight loss clinics found in shopping malls coast-to-coast and whose major concern lies in signing you up to buy a six months' supply of their company's prepackaged products. Independent dieticians are experts and can guide you toward a customized program that takes into account your specific needs and tastes.

Your dietician should discuss with you a wide assortment of foods that are low in fat, high in carbohydrates with moderate amounts of sugar, sodium, caffeine, and alcohol. A dietician should never make a medical diagnosis; he or she is only there to analyze your eating patterns and peculiarities. Be wary of any dietician who gives you a list of foods with very few options, unless you have a specific medical condition that precludes you from eating certain items. The number of daily calories should never be less than 1000—unless your physician has specifically prescribed such an approach.

What's more, be suspicious of any dietician who attempts to sell you a food supplement of any kind, such as vitamins or minerals. It's perfectly all right for a dietician to make a suggestion, but to offer any such substance for sale on the premises is not ethical. A dietician should be recommended through your doctor. If you don't have a doctor, call up your local hospital or community health center. They will most likely have an approved list.

If you wander through the Yellow Pages, avoid dieticians who advertise quick weight loss or imply they can cure you of any disease. Finally, when visiting a dietician, make sure the diet you receive is individually tailored for your needs; never accept a preprinted list of foods.

A Special Warning Sign

I've talked about too much body fat, but what happens if you really go overboard and wind up with too little? Well, that could be a problem as well, especially if you're in your twenties or thirties. Sometimes younger women who are endurance athletes, triathletes, or marathon runners lose so much body fat that they stop menstruating. Along with that, the supply of calcium and other minerals in their bones also depletes.

In fact, what happens is that you can have an incredibly in-shape athlete, maybe twenty-eight years old, who has the bone density of a sixty-year-old woman with osteoporosis. If she endures some slight injury, such as a tiny stress fracture, it can have devastating consequences because her bones are so weak. Therefore, it pays to be extremely cautious when training for endurance events. Always maintain the right amount of body fat.

In these types of activities a woman's body fat should essentially be 9 percent and a man's 3 percent. Anytime you start drifting below those levels, you're getting into an unhealthy range. So if you've been working out intensely and your period stops, that could be a warning sign requiring you to reassess your training priorities. Immediately go to a doctor to determine whether or not your percentage of body fat is below the essential limits.

CHAPTER 4

Developing Muscle Mass Without Becoming a Mass of Muscle

Many women are wary of training because they are worried about developing bulging muscles and appearing too masculine. They have visions of being transformed into a female version of Arnold Schwarzenegger. Well, I really have no intention of turning any woman into "The Terminator." In fact, even if you're a woman who tried her hardest to bulk up like my good friend Arnold, you could never come close.

This is due to testosterone, the active hormone found predominantly in males, which is needed for truly expanded muscular development. Over 99 percent of the women in the general population don't have anywhere near enough of this hormone to worry about developing explosive biceps and triceps.

From my experience, whenever women see their muscles tighten, they're probably witnessing changes they've never really seen before, so they automatically assume they're getting bigger in the arms, legs, or back. But what's happening is that they're actually firming up and losing inches. So this whole notion of growing larger is just an illusion.

The post-pregnancy training program is especially designed to help accentuate your curves. Perpetual problem spots such as hips, thighs, buns, and breasts all derive their shape from the muscles beneath. Therefore you have to concentrate on these muscle groups in order to rid yourself of flabby bulges. But don't worry—the effort will be well worth it.

Why Muscle Gives Off Good Vibes

The muscle fibers beneath your skin actually vibrate a slight amount twenty-four hours a day, whether you're awake or asleep, sitting or standing. This action alone differentiates them from bone and fat tissue, which are stagnant and literally just lie there. As your muscles grow, these oscillations allow you to eat more without putting on weight; because the muscle is constantly active, it needs to be fed. The more muscle, the more activity. The more calories expended, the more you can eat.

Even a moderate amount of added muscle will consume an extra 20 to 30 calories an hour. Do the math and you'll see there's potential to burn off an additional 720 calories a day. That's equivalent to a piece of cheesecake, two Milky Way candy bars, or an ice-cream cone with two scoops and sprinkles. Small wonder why world-renowned bodybuilders have to consume so much food. With their super physiques they burn as much as 55 to 75 calories more an hour than the regular person. Without pigging out, they'd literally starve.

How Gals Can Eat Just as Much as Guys

Up until now life has been unjust for women. But I don't mean just sexual harassment or other important rights issues. I mean that historically men have been able to eat more than women without putting on as much fat. Why this was so remained a total mystery until the advent of nutritional research to answer the question. Then it all became clear. Because of their higher levels of testosterone, a muscle-building hormone, men naturally burn off more calories. But thanks to advances in our understanding, women no longer have to be left behind in the fat-burning department. By firming up muscles, they can now virtually match men in this area, which means they can finally finish their meals without their husbands sticking their forks in.

Why Do Muscles Grow?

By lifting weights or doing any other kind of resistance exercise, such as chin-ups or sit-ups, you cause your muscles to contract. If the challenge is sufficiently great, your muscles rise to the occasion by synthesizing greater amounts of protein. As a consequence of all this straining, your muscle cells respond by expanding and growing stronger. Additionally, the connective tissue between your muscles and bones, the many tendons and ligaments, also become larger and more powerful during the process.

Challenging the outer limits of your strength will no doubt cause microscopic ruptures in the fibers of your ligaments and tendons as they try to adjust to the added strain. What's more, a small amount of swelling may also accompany these tiny rips. Both of these are the primary reasons for muscle soreness. But don't worry. These tears and swelling are a natural result of the opposing forces you put on your muscles, particularly during the stretch phase of an exercise when they have to lengthen to accommodate the weight, and then contract to achieve the flex.

> Don't get sore at your muscles for getting sore. Thank them instead, because sore muscles mean higher levels of fitness, a taut and slimmer body.

Even if you decide to take it easy at first, there's little you can do to avoid muscle soreness. So I don't recommend stopping your entire training program just because you experience a little soreness. This would be counterproductive. You simply have to work through the pain like any other barrier. Waiting for soreness to disappear will never lead to the results you want.

But here's the good news. While you can certainly anticipate a degree of discomfort the first week, this will gradually diminish through the second week and probably, by the end of the third week, disappear entirely. Just the process of training alone aids in healing all those anguished muscles because, as more blood is circulated through them, they become less constricted and tense. Which means you feel more re-laxed.

I Can't Take Any More

Oh, yes you can. I'm not going to let you off the hook that easily. If your muscles seem to be major disaster areas, soak yourself in a nice warm tub for about half an hour. Add some natural sea salts if you wish. But don't miss any workouts. Just lower the amount of weights you've been using or the level of aerobic exercise for about a week and then gradually bring it back up to the level where you were.

If you stop working out for a week, especially in the beginning, you'll discover that your body quickly retrogresses. Muscles and tendons lose elasticity. Then when you feel better and start training all over again, the soreness returns once more. I've seen the pattern over and over. And then folks really wind up sore at themselves.

When You're Really Injured, You'll Know It

Extreme soreness is one thing, but getting an honest to goodness injury is another. First of all there's nothing merely sore or "achy" about it. It's unusual to start feeling a serious injury the next day, since almost in-evitably you get whacked with the hurt immediately. And here I'm talk-ing sharp, shooting, wrenching, even excruciating pain that stops you dead in your tracks like a bolt of lightning.

By far, the most frequent types of injuries I see are fascia injuries—severe rips in the connective tissue that surrounds the muscle. Ligaments can also stretch and tear away from the bone. What's more, tendons can become inflamed, a condition better known as tendinitis. The bottom line is that all of these are serious conditions and may require a medical consultation before you proceed with your training.

Get to Know Your Muscles

1. THE BICEPS AND TRICEPS

Flexing the arm plus twisting the hand are the primary duties of the biceps muscles. Opposite the biceps on the back of the arm you'll find the triceps muscle. Chief responsibility for the triceps is moving the arm both away from and toward the body, as well as to extend the forearm. So by working the triceps and biceps, consider yourself fully armed.

2. THE DELTOIDS, LATISSIMUS DORSI, AND TRAPEZIUS

The deltoid muscles literally shoulder the load. A large and versatile muscle extending from the upper reaches of the shoulder blade across to the collarbone, its name derives from resembling the Greek letter delta since it's triangular in appearance. The deltoid works in close cooperation with its neighboring muscles. The anterior deltoid in partnership with the pectoral muscles help to raise the arm and extend it forward. Raising the arm sideways is the job of the medial deltoid. And lastly, the posterior deltoid unites with the latissimus dorsi to move the arm backward. The latissimus dorsi are the large muscles that run from the middle of your back to the tailbone. The "lats" work to pull the shoulders back and downward. Well-developed lats will help your waist appear smaller and minimize large hips. The trapezius muscle runs from the back of the neck to the middle of the back. It works to shrug the shoulders, pull the head and shoulders back, and when you raise anything above your head.

3. THE PECTORALIS MAJOR OR "PECS"

Stretching across the upper chest is the pectoralis major, also simply known as the pectorals. Starting at the collarbone, the pectorals extend beneath the chest and eventually wind up by the cartilage that attaches the upper ribs to the breastbone.

As a woman, your "pecs" are overshadowed by your breasts, which consist primarily of fatty tissue. By training the pectorals you can actually help uplift and shape your breasts so that they appear larger and fuller. On top of this, developing the pectorals will impart definition to the chest area or—nontechnically speaking—give you more cleavage.

4. THE ABDOMINALS

Most people find abdominal exercise the most abominable of all. An immensely powerful muscle, the rectus abdominous starts out from the rib cage and stretches vertically over the abdominal wall. While the rectus abdominous consists of only one elongated muscle, it often is referred to in the plural sense, because of its upper and lower sections, and because these are separately isolated during the course of working out.

Running diagonally to the rectus abdominous are the external oblique muscles. Together with other muscles these serve to rotate and bend the torso. Moving at right angles to the external obliques and just beneath them are the interior obliques. The shape of your waistline is derived from how these two muscle groups intersect with each other: the more diagonal the angle, the smaller your belt size.

5. THE HIPS AND BUTTOCKS MUSCLES

These are the muscles that are literally responsible for bringing up the rear. Three muscles are primarily responsible for the curvature of your butt: the gluteus maximus, which is the largest, the gluteus medius, and the gluteus minimis. The maximus's primary function is to rotate and position the thigh for heavy-duty work such as ascending stairs.

Below the maximus is the medius, whose duties include lifting the leg to one side plus keeping the hips in coordination and balance. Practically duplicating the tasks of the medius is the minimis. If you're confused by now, don't worry. The crucial thing is that each one of these muscles will be getting special attention during the post-pregnancy training.

6. THE FRONT, INNER, AND BACK LEG MUSCLES

I've saved the most complicated group for last, consisting of the quadriceps, sartorius, adductor, and biceps femoris or hamstring muscles. The quadriceps (which is actually four distinct muscles—hence the name) is used to raise your leg when you're sitting down.

Extending from the inner thigh to the back part of the knee is the sartorius. Primarily the sartorius is responsible for turning your thigh right and left. Also reaching from the inner thigh are the adductor muscles. Together with the other muscles in this area the adductors help contract, swivel, and pull the legs together when they're apart.

The gastrocnemius is a muscle in the calf of your leg. It helps bend the knee and flex the foot downward. We work this muscle when we run or do calf raises.

And last, but certainly not least, we have three muscles named the hamstrings. Beginning in the pelvis, all three of these muscles extend downward to the rear of the knee cap. One of the three, the biceps femoris, helps to bend the knee back and forth.

If you had a normal delivery, you can begin the post-pregnancy training about two weeks after giving birth. However, if there were complications, such as a cesarean, then you will have to wait about six to eight weeks before you can start. In any event, don't start my program before first determining your present level of fitness—as you will in chapter five.

CHAPTER 5

Evaluating Your Total Fitness

Each time I start working with a new client, we do a comprehensive workup of her fitness and medical history. My post-pregnancy training program pulls no punches, so having a complete understanding of each and every part of your body is absolutely vital for achieving the goals you desire. Your body is very much like a car. Preventative maintenance will go a long way to ensuring that it goes the distance it was intended to.

But like any vehicle, if you've been abusing it or you've been in an accident, there are obvious weak spots. You may not even be aware of them. It takes a series of trained observations to diagnose those vulnerable points and then get them up to maximum efficiency. They say a chain is only as strong as its weakest link. As a personal trainer, I make sure that every link in your body pulls its own weight.

I always work in conjunction with the advice of a doctor and have a rule of thumb regarding my clients. For those under thirty, and if a checkup within the past year has revealed no serious health problems, then it is okay for them to begin my training program. I insist that clients between thirty and thirty-nine be examined by a doctor no later than three months before starting my exercise regimen, and during this time they should also have an electrocardiogram (ECG) taken at rest.

Those between forty and fifty-nine, especially if they've been sedentary for a long period of time, should observe the same procedures as the thirty to thirty-nine group with one additional test—an ECG taken during exercising, also commonly called a treadmill or cardiac stress test. Those over fifty-nine years of age should follow the same guidelines as the 40 to 59 group, except that it's important for them to have their medical exam performed right away, before they embark on the training program.

But before moving on, answer the followings questions:

General Health Appraisal

1. Have you ever been diagnosed as having any type of heart trouble?
2. Have you ever experienced pains in your heart or chest during exercising, afterward, or at other times?
3. Did either of your parents die from a heart attack before the age of sixty?
4. Have you periodically felt faint or suffered from dizzy spells?
5. Has your blood pressure ever been monitored as being too high? Too low?
6. Has a qualified medical professional ever informed you that you have a bone or joint problem, such as arthritis, which may be compounded by engaging in a workout program?
7. Is low back pain a chronic condition?
8. Have you ever been treated for serious illnesses of the lungs, such as chronic bronchitis or emphysema?
9. Have you ever suffered any major bodily injuries in an accident?
10. Would you classify yourself as an alcohol abuser?
11. Are you addicted to any drugs?
12. Do you regularly take tranquilizers or sleeping pills?
13. Have you ever been or are you now a smoker?
14. Has anyone in your immediate family ever had diabetes?
15. Have you ever been treated for diseases of the kidneys, thyroid, or liver?
16. Have you ever had any type of rectal growth or bleeding (other than hemorrhoids)?
17. Do you suffer from frequent migraines?
18. Have you ever undergone radiation or chemotherapy?
19. Do you currently have any sort of physical disability which interferes with normal movement?
20. Would you classify yourself as obese (men: 25 percent over recommended weight; women: 30 percent over recommended weight)?
21. Do you suffer from any serious gastrointestinal problems (such as colitis or ulcers)?

22. Has your mother, sister, or daughter ever had breast cancer?
23. Were the results of your last Pap smear abnormal?
24. Do you experience unusually heavy vaginal bleeding?

Answering "no" to the above questions suggest that you are in relatively good shape. However, no matter what your age group, if the response was "yes" to any of the above, then you should immediately have a medical checkup before starting my post-pregnancy program. This exam should always include an examination of your heart, blood vessels, joints, and muscles.

You should also be told your blood pressure. Two numbers make up this reading. The first is *systolic* pressure, and it determines the degree of pressure in your arteries just after your heart has pumped. The second is called *diastolic* pressure, which measures the pressure in the arteries between beats, when your heart is relaxed. By putting these two numbers together you get your total blood pressure, such as 120/70. Current medical standards point to 120/80 as the ideal reading.

Nevertheless, even one as low as 90/70 is usually no cause for alarm. But a measurement over 140/90 may suggest a problem. Even so, don't hit the panic button. To get a confirmed diagnosis of high blood pressure you must have it taken a number of times. Outside influences (for instance stress or even diet) can easily alter your blood pressure readings.

On the Level About Cholesterol

What's more, a blood test should be done to measure your cholesterol levels, which is important, because it's a precise indication of the amount of fat in your blood. The majority of the medical community agrees that any cholesterol under 200 is acceptable while a range of between 150 and 180 is desirable. That figure is then broken down into the three basic components of cholesterol. But here I'm concerned with just two of them: HDL (High-Density Lipoprotein) and LDL (Low-Density Lipoprotein).

So what does this all mean? Very simply, the higher the reading for your HDL, the healthier you are likely to be. But with LDL it's just the opposite: The lower the measure, the luckier you are. For HDL a range of 30 to 80 is about normal, with numbers over 50 considered to be optimal. On the other hand, the average range for LDL is 80 to 185, although to be considered in the good category, you must be under a 100.

Perhaps the most important figure is your Total Cholesterol/HDL ratio, which, as the name suggests, is your cholesterol count divided by your HDL. For example, if your total cholesterol is 168 and your HDL is 42, then the radio is 4:1. Healthy males usually score 4:1 to 5:1, with the average woman ranging between 4:1 to 4.5:1. If you're wondering about heart disease, a ratio under 3.5:1 for men and 3.2:1 for women puts you in the lowest risk group.

One more test I suggest is a glucose readup. This determines the amount of sugar in your blood. It's an early test for diabetes and a crucial figure to know.

If you're already reading this section, then I assume there's no medical problem serious enough after your pregnancy to keep you from meeting the minimum requirements for this workout. But just as it doesn't take an auto mechanic to spot a car that needs a new exhaust system or whose chassy has been dented, it doesn't take a trained professional to assess your overall physical condition. In fact, you can do it yourself.

Each day of your life three vital areas of fitness are being unofficially measured dozens of times. These reflect your aerobic state of conditioning, general strength, as well as your body's flexibility. One of the immediate joys of starting an exercise program is feeling the dramatic improvement in just performing everyday jobs and maneuvers. The following list of activities—or their equivalents—will reveal whether or not your body is operating at its most ideal level.

Everyday Aerobic Condition Indicators

- When you climb up several flights of stairs, do you find yourself sweating and winded with your heart pounding in your chest?
- Have you ever felt faint while simply walking at higher elevations? (Altitude can very often reveal problems with your level of fitness.)
- Can you shovel snow for more than twenty minutes without having to take a break?

- Have you ever strolled through the city of San Francisco, or any other hilly location, and experienced soreness in your calves or ankle pain?
- Can you dance to rock, Latin, or disco rhythms for at least half an hour without feeling like collapsing?
- Could you run to catch a train or bus and not be concerned about having a heart attack?
- Are you capable of making love without having to catch your breath every couple of minutes?

Everyday Strength Indicators

Besides your aerobic condition, another area that greatly affects your everyday sense of well-being is your strength. Just how strong are you? How strong would you like to be? Again, much is revealed by commonplace activities. If none of the following specifically apply to your life, then substitute something equivalent which you might have to perform.

- Would you be able to lift a twenty-pound sack of kitty litter or a box of books with both hands? What about one hand?
- Do you ever move around the furniture where you live? What about tables, desks, or bookshelves?
- Are you able to lift a two-year-old child off the ground? What about a five-year-old? Could you carry a ten-year-old across the backyard?
- Would you be able to hammer twelve two-inch nails into a piece of plywood without your arm going limp?
- Could you break a wooden ruler in half using both hands?
- Without using hot water or a hammer, can you unscrew the lid off a jar of jelly that's stuck?
- Would you be capable of picking up your mattress and flipping it over to the other side?
- If you were locked out of your house, could you climb up fifteen feet to an open window?

Everyday Flexibility Indicators

Together with strength and aerobic fitness, flexibility is crucial in designing a workout program that's perfect for you. Flexibility is a key benefit of the post-pregnancy training. By being flexible your body can bend where it would otherwise break. You appear more graceful and slender, moving with ease at every turn.

It's vital to understand how flexible you are before you begin my program because your body's capacity to be limber and pliable reveals much about your present fitness level. A certain amount of flexibility is required to perform nearly all of the exercises coming up, so before we start I will be focusing on how to stretch properly as well.

Symmetry and balance are essential parts of flexibility. Often because of old injuries or physical weaknesses, women tend to favor one part of their bodies over another. For instance, you may be able to touch your head to your knee on the right side but not on your left. If not corrected, performing exercise routines asymmetrically can lead to serious consequences. Following are ways of determining your body's flexibility.

- When putting on a bra, are you able to fasten it in back of you?
- Could you tie your shoes while standing up and without bending your knees?
- Is it easy for you to scratch your back? What about between the shoulder blades?
- Are you capable of stretching up and replacing a lightbulb that's several feet above your head?
- Without using your hands for support, could you comfortably crouch a full two minutes while waiting to surprise someone?
- With your knees flat on the floor, are you able to sit with your buttocks on your heels?
- Can you look over your right and left shoulder just by turning your head around?
- If you had to climb over a fence half your height, could you make it by swinging one foot across the top and then the other to reach the other side?

The Three Crucial Fitness Areas

Obviously, the more of these tasks that you can easily perform, the better your fitness level. However, before you can arrive at where you're going, you first have to know precisely where you are. Having an accurate picture of your present fitness level can help accelerate your progress, while decreasing the possibility of any pitfalls during your workout program.

There are a number of specific areas that must be evaluated after giving birth, but first I'm going to concentrate on the three we touched on right above: your aerobic condition, muscle strength, and flexibility.

The measure of aerobic fitness determines how well your body converts oxygen to energy. Simply put, the healthier your cardiovascular system, the more capable you are of generating the power needed to achieve your workout goals. The key significance of aerobic conditioning is that it strengthens your heart, allowing it to function with greater ease while still delivering all the energy your body requires.

As you reach premium aerobic fitness, your heart starts to beat more slowly—both at rest and during exercise—and this can measurably improve your life expectancy. Just like any other mechanical pump, the less the heart has to work, the less strain you put on it, the more likely it will last without difficulty or breakdown. Slowing down your pulse will be a critical element of your workout, until we reach your ideal heart rate.

The first series of aerobic tests requires little more than a stopwatch. You can buy a cheap digital version for only a few dollars. Setting your goals depends on your initial scores, so don't overlook this part of your total training program.

A word of caution: If you experience severe shortness of breath, nausea, dizziness, or lightheadedness from any of these tests or feel you can't continue, then stop immediately. Have a doctor evaluate your medical condition before continuing this workout.

The One-Mile Clocked Walk

This is probably the most basic aerobic test you can take, as walking is the most accessible of all exercises. The best place to try this is at your local high school athletic track. Make sure to determine the circumference of the track so that you can see how many trips around will be required. If no running track is available, simply use a flat street or roadway with minimal cross traffic.

Time (in minutes and seconds)	Aerobic Rating
11:30 or under	Terrific!
11:41 to 13:05	Very Superior
13:06 to 14:35	Pretty Good
14:36 to 16:05	Average
16:06 to 17:35	Just Fair
17:36 and above	Poor

The Mile and a Half Clocked Jog

If you're already involved with running, active in some other aerobic program, or play sports such as tennis or racquetball, then this test will give you a better picture of your present level of fitness than just walking alone. It also provides you with an indicator of muscle strength. This is particularly true for swimmers, who aerobically may be in fine shape, but who sometimes lack resilience in their legs when they're on dry ground.

Age:		18–30	31–40	41–50	51–60
Fitness Level 1: *Superb*	TIME:	12:30 or less	13:00 or less	13:45 or less	14:30 or less
Fitness Level 2: *Excellent*	TIME:	12:31–13:30	13:01–14:30	13:46–15:55	14:31–16:30
Fitness Level 3: *Very Good*	TIME:	13:31–15:54	14:31–16:30	15:56–17:30	16:31–19:00
Fitness Level 4: *About Average*	TIME:	15:55–18:30	16:31–19:00	17:31–19:30	19:01–20:00
Fitness Level 5: *Only Fair*	TIME:	18:31–20:30	19:01–21:30	19:31–23:30	20:01–25:00
Fitness Level 6: *Poor*	TIME:	20:31/plus	21:31/plus	23:31/plus	25:00/plus

Evaluating Joint and Muscular Condition

The number-one rule concerning joints and muscles is that you shouldn't be aware of them. Unless you heavily overexert yourself, there should be little muscle soreness. Likewise, your joints should move easily with no grinding or discomfort. Obviously there are chronic conditions such as arthritis which affect the functioning of our body mechanisms. The following section will help you pinpoint joint and muscle weakness.

Are there weak points in your body? Places where you experience frequent pain or swelling? Do you hesitate to engage in certain sports or activities because of fear of injury? Again, these can all affect a balanced post-pregnancy fitness program. Prompted by such concerns, you might neglect to work one area while totally overdoing another. **If a serious injury or weakness prevents you from doing any type of exercise, make sure to consult with a qualified doctor to find out the best way to compensate for it.**

Knees: The Number-One Injury

The numbers prove it. The knee is the joint in your body most vulnerable to sports and fitness injuries. In fact more than 25 percent of all fitness injuries involve the knee, not to mention a whopping 75 percent of all surgery. Among those involved in a regular workout program, joggers have the highest percentage of knee injuries. Not too far behind are those millions of men and women who participate in aerobic dancing of one sort or another. Even swimmers aren't immune to this type of injury, especially those who prefer the breaststroke, for as they thrust through the water, undue strain can be put on the knee joint.

Knee difficulties usually stem from a previous injury that traumatized ligaments, cartilage, or tendons. Although these always require special attention during the healing process, many times people overlook fully rehabilitating their knees by strengthening the surrounding muscles.

> After any knee injury, don't be hasty about returning to a full-fledged workout program. A second injury more serious than the first may occur—and could be that much harder to repair.

If a knee injury has required surgery, particularly where a cast was involved, then premature wearing down of the joint, which is known as arthritis, becomes a real factor. You must be aware that more than half of all knee injuries can eventually lead to arthritis. Initial symptoms include aching and grinding in the knee joints, locking or swelling, plus a decrease in flexibility.

The quadriceps muscle, the large muscles that run up and down the front of the thigh and particularly the small section called the vastus medialis, which is located just above and toward the inside of the kneecap, has the job of making sure that your knee functions properly. If there's weakness in the quadriceps and you put too much strain on the area, then the whole knee can buckle, resulting in an unpleasant number of side effects.

To assist in avoiding knee injuries I've developed special exercises to strengthen and develop the quadriceps muscles. But before we delve into any of these, I want to first diagnose the condition of your knees. In order to get the best results from your training program, the knees, as well as every other part of your body, must operate in balance and harmony. We'll start with the most serious questions first.

Evaluating the Fitness of Your Knees

Important: Make sure that you evaluate both your right and left knee. This will determine which one is stronger and which one is weaker, if such is the case.

KNEE EXAM #1

1. At any time has a trained medical professional advised you to wear a knee brace?
2. Are there moments when you suspect that your knee is "loose"?
3. Have you ever experienced your knee buckling, failing, or locking in any way?
4. When engaging in any form of physical exertion, do your knees have a tendency to swell up?

Should any of these questions elicit a "yes" answer, then you probably have a knee condition serious enough to warrant immediate medical attention. Do not engage in any training program until you have consulted a physician. However, if you responded "no" to each one, then move on and see how you respond to the following:

KNEE EXAM #2

1. Have you noticed that your knee hurts when either climbing up or down inclines such as hills?
2. When sitting down for two or three hours with your knees bent, is there any stiffness or pain when you get up?
3. Are there any times when you experience being "weak at the knees," as if they were going to go out from under you?

All of the above indicate early stages of more damaging conditions. The good news is that most of these problems can most likely be corrected by strengthening the muscles in your leg, as well as by determining which knee is causing the other to strain or compensate.

In the next section you'll find out if both your knees are working in perfect unison. Even those in good condition may discover subtle differences in the performance of each knee. Nevertheless, it's good to catch them early on, before they pose a risk to your training program.

KNEE EXAM #3

1. Sit on the floor with your legs straight out in front of you. Observe the shallow indentations on either side of your kneecaps. Are these depressions of equal size and depth?
2. Remain on the floor. Examine the large muscles in the front of your thighs. These are the quadriceps. Just over your kneecap toward the inside lies the vastus medialis. Now tense these muscles and compare them. Are both the right and the left the same size? Are both quadriceps equally hard?
3. While lying flat on your stomach, bend your knees back as much as they will go. Turn your head around and take a look. Are both heels the same distance from your rear end?
4. This next evaluation requires a knee extension machine. You can find one at any gym. With one leg and then the other, try to lift at least fifteen percent of your total body weight. Were you able to do equally well on both sides? (NOTE: It's self-defeating to raise the weight with both legs. For example, if you raised eighty

pounds, you might assume that each leg can handle forty, without realizing the stronger leg is doing most of the lifting.)

If you answered "no" to any of these, this indicates either one or both your legs are not as strong as they should be. Ideally speaking, both the right and left knee should be equivalent in terms of strength and flexibility. If they are, then you can proceed to any exercises in the training program that involve using the knees. However, should one knee be weaker or more painful than the other, then we will have to make adjustments. I suggest doing an extra set of leg extensions (see page 150), but using only the weak leg.

If you experience any pain, swelling, or weakness in your knees, I recommend that you cut down on activities that aggravate the situation. For instance, substitute cycling for jogging or use a stair climber instead of taking a step class. If you don't want to substitute, at least alternate activities.

No-no's for Knee Injuries

1. Knee extensions with too many pounds of weight.
2. Jogging or any exercise utilizing a treadmill.
3. Stair climbers or step workouts.
4. Lunges or squats.
5. Using a rowing machine with knees bent more than 90 degrees.
6. Stationary or regular bicycling where the seat is set too low.

Evaluating the Fitness of Your Back

Lower back pain afflicts just about all of us at some point in our lives, especially during and after pregnancy, and you're probably no exception. Most times back problems are relatively benign and are caused by overexertion, such as trying to move a box that's too heavy, overdoing it while planting in the garden, or attempting to lift a heavy suitcase off an airport carousel.

In and of itself, minor back pain shouldn't discourage you from engaging in a personal training program. As a matter of fact, physicians who specialize in sports medicine often recommend a complete exercise regimen as a way of preventing and treating common back problems. On the other hand, problems of the more serious variety can be quite agonizing and debilitating—for no other injury can so completely incapacitate a person as a back mishap.

Besides knocking you down flat, back injuries can be highly dangerous, particularly when they involve the backbone or the spinal cord lying underneath. Since the spinal cord is the brain's information superhighway to the rest of the body, any trauma can interfere with the overall nervous system. In the worst case scenario, spinal column damage can result in paralysis.

But as I mentioned, the vast majority of back problems are *not* dangerous. The most cost-effect way of treating all the chronic aches and stiffness is through simple prevention. In other words, you have to learn how to strengthen the muscles in your back and make them more flexible. Let's do an initial workup on the current shape of your back.

BACK EXAM #1

1. Have you ever experienced pain radiating down either or both of your legs?
2. Are there times while coughing, sneezing, or straining on the toilet that you are stricken with back pain or pain radiating through your arms or legs?
3. Is it difficult for you to muster enough strength to stand on your toes?
4. Have you periodically encountered sensations of numbness or tingling in one or both of your feet or legs?
5. In the past two years, have you been immobilized due to extreme back pain or trauma to your back, such as a sports injury or car accident?
6. Has a medical diagnosis, including X rays, ever shown that you have a ruptured disk or any other type of spinal deterioration?

An answer of "yes" to just one of these questions may indicate a serious underlying back condition. Therefore, before starting an exercise program, you should consult a doctor to see if there are any limitations that have to be placed on your workout. However, if your response was negative to all the above questions, then we can move on to the next series.

BACK EXAM #2

1. Upon awakening in the morning, do you ever notice that your back is stiff?
2. When you've been sitting or standing for twenty minutes or more, do you experience pains in your back?
3. If you sporadically engage in certain forms of exertion, such as tennis, golf, softball, or even dancing, does your back ache the day afterward?

A "yes" answer to any of these questions indicates you'll have to pay special attention to the care of your back as the post-pregnancy training commences. One of the best back strengthening exercises is the second cool down stretch for the lower back that appears on page 105. It is also known as the cobra stretch. I recommend doing this stretch every day if you have any form of back pain.

By answering "no" to the above questions, you've demonstrated that your back is in fairly good condition. Just to be absolutely certain, however, I recommend going on to the third section of this evaluation.

BACK EXAM #3

1. While sitting on the floor, stretch your legs straight out in front of you. Are you able to effortlessly extend your fingers beyond your kneecaps?
2. Stretch out on your stomach with your forehead and toes touching the floor. Can you lift your legs off the floor, while at the same time arching your chest upward so that you're totally supported by your stomach? Is the effort painless?
3. Are you easily able to bend in all four directions? Forward? Backward? Over to the right? Over to the left? Can you perform the same motions with your arms stretched above your head?
4. With your feet planted straight forward can you twist a full 90 degrees to the right? Now can you do it to the left?

If you passed all three sections, you are ready to begin a workout program that fully incorporates the back. But if a few areas are sensitive, you should pay attention to the following:

No-no's for Back Injuries:

1. Reaching down and attempting to touch your toes.
2. Excessively stretching the hamstring muscles.
3. Overburdening yourself while lifting weights.
4. Doing sit-ups with feet anchored under any stationary support.

Evaluating the Fitness of Your Ankles

Your ankles are the crucial link between your legs and your feet. Hence they bear the brunt of many quick twists and turns as you exercise. These occasionally cause ankle sprains, one of the most widespread sports injuries.

A minor sprain that causes you to hobble around for a day or two is rarely anything to worry about. It's the more debilitating type that causes concern. A sprain requiring being on crutches for more than a week, wearing a cast, or which resulted in surgery may cause complications in the future such as weakness, pain, swelling, and recurrent injuries.

Ankle Exam #1

1. Are you experiencing sharp, knifelike pains in your ankles that have no obvious cause?
2. Have your ankles a history of locking or catching, needing movements such as a turning or jiggling to fix the problem?
3. Are your ankles prone to giving way or even collapsing, which later results in swelling?
4. With both feet flat on the floor, examine your ankles by sitting down in front of a mirror. Is either one more pronounced than the other? More swollen? Much bigger? Deformed?

Answering "yes" to any of the preceding questions may indicate a serious problem with your ankles. Before starting any training program I would strongly advise that you seek medical advice. You could have a condition that would be difficult or impossible to remedy on your own. However, if none of the above is a concern, then go on to the next series of questions.

ANKLE EXAM #2

1. Do your ankles wind up being twisted or sprained twice a year or more?
2. Will your ankles be stiff the day after strenuous activity?
3. While walking over uneven ground does your ankle sometimes fail to adjust adequately, making you lose your balance?

While a "yes" answer to any of the above shouldn't cause too much anxiety, to avoid injury make sure you wear well-made workout shoes with good ankle support, while we work on strengthening your ankles. But if your answer was "no" to all of the preceding questions, then in all likelihood your ankles are in fine condition. However, to be completely assured, pay attention to the next part.

ANKLE EXAM #3

1. Stand in front of a full-length mirror. Now turn completely around so that your back faces it. Stand up on your toes as far as you can go. Look over your shoulder and observe the reflection of your calves. Is one smaller or less muscular than the other?
2. Sit down in a comfortable chair. Extend your legs straight out with your heels touching the floor. Point your toes as much as you can. Do you notice that one set of toes is bending farther down than the other ones?
3. Face a wall and stand about two feet away. Put both hands flat against it and lean forward, making sure your legs are only an inch from each other and that your knees are straight. Is there discomfort or pain in either the right or left ankle?
4. Clasp your hands straight in front of you for balance. Then, with your feet parallel and flat on the floor, squat down as deeply as you can. Is one ankle unable to go as far down as the other?

Answering "no" to all these questions means your ankles are in optimum condition and that you are ready to begin a post-pregnancy fitness program. If the answer to any of them was "yes," then be aware that you might still be having trouble with the effects of a previous ankle injury. Be aware that some forms of aerobic exercises will be preferable to others.

These include rowing, cycling, and swimming. Others should be avoided because they might easily cause reinjury.

No-no's for Ankle Injuries:

1. Aerobic Dancing
2. Tennis
3. Jogging
4. Racquetball
5. Step Training

Evaluating the Fitness of Your Shoulders

When using free weights or machines for toning and creating muscle definition, the shoulders are a crucial area and focus point. Now while the shoulder is the most flexible joint in your whole body, paradoxically it's also the most likely to require tightening and adjustment.

Most of your other joints, such as in the ankle or knee, are bound together firmly by a series of tough ligaments. However, in order to keep moving in a loose, circular direction, the shoulder relies on well-coordinated muscles and tendons to keep it functioning. And therein lies the problem. If your shoulder muscles are not up to doing the job, it can disrupt your overall balance and thereby become a real physical problem down the line.

Unfortunately, shoulder weakness is one of the most difficult to detect. This is because your shoulders often seem to accomplish the daily chores of life with little or no difficulty, so scant attention is paid to them. In fact, you might unconsciously avoid using your shoulders in any way that causes discomfort. For example, you may chronically hunch over if raising your shoulders up straight causes pain. In other instances, say when reaching for an object lying on a shelf above your head, you may favor the shoulder that gives you the most trouble and use the other.

To train successfully, a healthy pair of shoulders is an absolute must. Check and see if yours are operating at the optimum level.

Shoulder Exam #1

1. Is either of your shoulders unstable? Subject to slipping out of position, discoloration, or dislocation?

2. Has either one of your shoulders a tendency to lock, catch, or become frozen in one position?
3. Have you experienced sensations of numbness or tingling moving down along your arm into your hand? What about a sudden weakness in those areas?

Answering "yes" to any one of the previous questions may indicate a serious shoulder condition, one that requires prompt medical attention. But if none of the above is an issue, then move along to the next series of questions.

SHOULDER EXAM #2

1. Is there ever pain or stiffness in one shoulder, and not the other, particularly after exerting yourself?
2. When it comes to carrying hefty objects, such as strapping a large suitcase across your shoulder, is there one shoulder weaker than the other? One shoulder you avoid using altogether?
3. Gaze into a mirror with your arms straight down your sides. Now imagine a line going across the top of your collarbone. Against this line, check to see if your shoulders are the same height. Is one slumping lower than the other?

An answer of "yes" to any of these questions means that the strength in your shoulders has to be equalized. In the course of training you will be building up your shoulder muscles, and over time their strength will equalize. The power pivot and arm circle exercises that appear on page 156 are especially good for strengthening the shoulders.

SHOULDER EXAM #3

1. Gaze into the mirror with your arms resting flat against your sides. Now raise them slowly until they're both at a 45 degree angle to your body. As you perform this, does one shoulder come up higher?
2. Stand up straight, legs close together, and then slowly extend your arms out from your sides. Start raising them upward and then touch your fingertips over the middle of your head. Still in the air, turn your arms around so that the palms of your hands are now

touching. Is it more difficult to perform this maneuver with one arm than the other?

3. Find a comfortable place to lie down on your back. Have your arms stretched out away from you and touching the floor. Now bend your elbows until a right angle is formed, with the top of your hands toward your shoulders. Slowly allow them to descend until the top of your hands touch the floor in back of your head. Does one hand drop more easily than the other? Is there one hand that cannot reach the floor at all?

If none of the preceding presented any difficulty, then you are ready to engage in a full weight-lifting and body-sculpting program. However, answering "yes" to any of the above questions shows that one shoulder is weaker than the other. To protect the weaker shoulder, be aware of the following:

No-no's for Shoulder Injuries

1. Excessive weight lifting that puts undue strain on the shoulder
2. Nordic Track
3. Cross-country skiing
4. Any form of push-ups or chin-ups
5. Strenuous activities involving the shoulder: the breaststroke while swimming, golf, tennis, or basketball.

CHAPTER 6

Definitions to Give Your Body Definition

Let's start with the definition of *definition*. Definition is the quality of accenting and bringing out lines of muscle. As you do the post-pregnancy training, you will begin seeing in only a matter of months lines of definition, especially in your shoulders and upper back area. Definition is a key ingredient of body sculpting. Each area should be fully delineated and distinctive, with no overlapping or asymmetry to distract the eye. Here are some additional terms I will be using throughout the training.

Aerobic: Exercises that concentrate on your heart, lungs, and circulatory system.

Agonist: Any muscle that contracts and produces force.

Anabolic: Promoting or increasing growth, particularly of muscles.

Anaerobic: An exercise that takes place within a relatively short burst and that doesn't utilize oxygen as an energy source. In addition it doesn't elevate the heart rate over a long period of time. For example: powerlifting.

Antagonist: The name of the muscle that relaxes when the agonist (the opposing muscle) is working.

Atrophy: When a muscle shrinks in size, usually from lack of use.

Bar: The metal shaft of a barbell. They are usually one inch in diameter and encased in a revolving sleeve.

Barbell: A basic piece of weight-training equipment consisting of a bar that joins a sleeve, weight plates, and collars.

Buffed: Looking good or in great shape, especially as it relates to muscle tone and development.

Burn: The warm feeling a muscle has when it has been pushed to the limit.

Carbo Loading: Saturating your body with carbohydrates before an exceptionally grueling exercise, such as a marathon.

Cardiovascular Workout: Same as aerobic exercise.

Circuit Training: A group of related exercises performed one after another with no rest in between.

Collar: A metal clamp used to fasten weight plates onto a barbell.

Contraction: The period when the muscle fibers shorten, producing the force needed to lift weight or move bones.

Cooldown Period: Small movements accompanied by moderate stretching after working out. Useful for getting the heart rate back to normal, as well as preventing blood from gathering within the legs.

Definition: Muscle development without the appearance of fat.

Density: The relative hardness and thickness of your muscles. If a muscle is hard, it has density. The more effort you put into eliminating body fat, and the more strenuously you exercise, the more density your muscles will exhibit.

Dumbbell: A fixed weight joined to a small metal bar that's used in either hand during exercising.

Duration: The total time you spend on each activity, such as thirty minutes of jogging.

Endorphins: Powerful hormones that the pituitary gland secretes during endurance exercises; they have the effect of producing a natural feeling of peace and well-being.

Essential Fat: The fat you *don't* want to lose. It's critical to body function and no diet or exercise program should deplete this reserve of energy.

Extension: After flexing a muscle, this is the process of moving your limbs or body back to a normal stance.

Flex: Displaying your muscle by contracting it tightly.

Flexibility: Your overall range of motion within your joints, determined primarily by your tendons and ligaments.

Forced Reps: With the help of a partner, the last couple of repetitions within a set.

Free Weights: Refers most often to barbells and dumbbells, as opposed to workout machines, such as the Nautilus or Universal variety, that you commonly find in health clubs.

Frequency: The number of times a week you will be performing a particular exercise.

Hyperplasia: Technical term that explains muscle growth through the tearing of microscopic fibers.

Intensity: How much effort you put forth. The amount of weight you train with as compared to the number of pounds you can lift.

Intervals: Exercising in specific segments or portions.

Isolation Exercises: Special positions in which you compel your muscle to work harder by countering the force of gravity.

Kinesiology: Scientific research into human movement.

Lats: Short for latissimus muscles, which define the upper back.

LBM: Lean Body Mass. A percentage derived from the difference between muscle and fat tissue.

Lifting Belt: For those who want to tackle heavy weights and avoid injury, a leather belt fastened tightly around the waist.

Ligament: A tough form of fibrous tissue that connects bones to bones or bones to joints.

LSD: Long Slow Distances; the difference between aerobic jogging at a moderate speed and sprinting, which is usually anaerobic.

Maximum Oxygen Uptake: The body's capacity to metabolize oxygen into energy. The people with the highest uptakes are marathon runners and cross-country skiers.

Mode: The specific type of exercise you're doing, such as cycling, weight lifting, swimming, etc.

Muscle Mass: The true size of a muscle, as measured by length, width, and depth. Muscle mass is increased the more you train; therefore, it has greater volume. This process of muscle growth is called *hypertrophy*.

Muscle Pull: A colloquialism for a strain or a slight muscle tear, usually in the vicinity of the tendon or ligament.

Muscularity: This indicates the amount of muscle in relation to fat tissue. As you continue working out, the percentage of muscle to fat increase, and hence your muscularity. Also the dimension and definition of all the body's muscle groups considered together.

Myofibril: The actual muscle fiber itself. Each individual muscle comprises millions of them.

Overload: Adding additional pounds to the weight you lift, making the exercise routine tougher.

Pecs: Short for pectoral muscles, which stretch across the upper chest.

Plateau: The level of conditioning you reach where you have to step up the intensity of the workout in order to maintain your target heart rate.

Plates: Circular weights of various poundage which can be fastened onto a barbell.

Poundage: The amount of weight on a barbell or dumbbell.

PRE: Progressive Resistance Exercise. This refers to the adding of weight to specific exercises over time when the weights being used for the exercises are no longer enough of a challenge.

Proportion: The balanced development of symmetrical muscle groups.

Push/Pull Workout: Coordinating muscle groups that "push," such as the triceps, deltoids, and pectorals, with the ones that "pull," such as the lats and biceps.

Quads: Short for the quadriceps, muscles that run along the front of the thigh.

Red Muscle Fiber: Popularly called slow-twitch fiber, this is actually the endurance part of the muscle that is designed to fatigue slowly.

Rep: Abbreviation for *repetition*. The act of performing one complete motion of a particular exercise.

Resistance: As with poundage, the actual weight used while performing an exercise.

Rest Period: How much time is taken to relax between exercises.

"Ripped" Muscle: This is a muscle that has maximum definition, so much so that it appears striated or "ripped." This ripple effect can be seen on bodybuilders who have taken extreme pains to develop every one of their muscle groups, particularly the abdominals, chest, and shoulders.

ROM: Range of motion within your joints; the amount of flexibility you have.

Set: A group of repetitions.

Split Workouts: Exercising the upper portion of your body on one training day, and the lower part the next.

Spot Reduction: The myth that you can remove fat from one area without affecting the fat everywhere.

Stretching: Positioning your body's limbs in such a way as to exceed the "comfort zone" of your muscles and lengthen connective tissue.

Striation: An extreme form of definition in which muscles and connective fibers literally seem to pop out from under the skin.

Supersets: Doing a set of one exercise, immediately followed by another. These are usually performed to develop antagonistic muscle groups.

Symmetry: Keeping your physical development in proportion so that each muscle in your body perfectly compliments all the rest, achieving a true sense of beauty and aesthetic balance.

Tendon: An exceptionally strong and pliant form of tissue that adheres the muscle to the bone.

Tension: The amount of power exerted when a muscle contracts.

Valsalva: The very serious mistake of holding your breath as you exert yourself, particularly when lifting weights. This unconscious action can cause pulmonary as well as other forms of internal injury. Under no circumstances should you stop inhaling and exhaling as you work out.

Vascularity: Veins that often become plainly displayed due to ultra low-body fat and dehydration.

Volume: How much "work" you actually put into your workout, the total amount of exercises, including sets, reps, and aerobic conditioning.

Warm-up: A crucial part of training not to be skipped. Stretching, mild calisthenics or any other kind of exercise designed specifically to ready tissue and raise the heart rate in preparation for the more strenuous part of your workout.

Weight Training: Has come to mean the same as "pumping iron."

White Muscle Fiber: The fibers that produce a sudden burst of power. Also known as fast-twitch fiber, they contract and tire quickly.

Working to Failure: Pushing muscles to complete fatigue by performing reps until they literally can contract no more.

CHAPTER 7

The Absolute Essentials of Working Out

Incredible results are what this post-pregnancy training is all about, the total and astonishing transformation of your health and appearance. But as all worthwhile things in life, these are not handed to you on a silver platter. If you want to get into the best shape possible, then you have to take the best possible approach. It's as simple as that. There are no quickie fixes, no gimmicks, no shortcuts in my program. You're getting the same guidance I give all my clients.

What Kind of Equipment?

First of all you don't have to belong to a gym in order to do the post-pregnancy training. Most of the exercises can be done at home with very little equipment—which makes them exceptionally convenient. I have nothing against gyms, but they can be a bit intimidating, especially if you're a little out-of-shape after giving birth. Walking, running, biking, hiking, using dumbbells—these are all easy to master with relative privacy.

Picture Perfect

During the post-pregnancy training, you're going to start a photo gallery, except you'll be the only one in the pictures. I find nothing helps motivation more than before and after photos while working out. That's why before you commence, you're going to take pictures of yourself or have someone else take pictures of you: full-length, front, back, plus closeups of the stomach, thighs, chest, and buttocks.

I recommend taking a set of photos every couple of weeks. Naturally, it's best to do this while wearing a bathing suit.

If your commitment ever falters, pull out the pictures from the weeks or months before and compare all the differences. They'll be pretty apparent. The major trouble with working out is that you soon forget where you started. You fail to realize all the progress you've made in a relatively short period of time. The familiar cliché is absolutely true. When it comes to motivating yourself, pictures are worth a thousand words.

Aerobic or Anaerobic? That Is the Question

I see a lot of people running every day who still don't have the type of muscle mass or amount of definition they should. Without a doubt these are individuals who are constantly training—but just aerobically. They're simply not supplementing their training program with anaerobic strength workouts.

In spite of their smashing cardiovascular systems, many of them have loose, flabby areas, particularly around their stomachs and upper arms. Proper weight training would tighten up those problem spots. Hence, it's imperative to exercise both aerobically and anaerobically, not just substitute one for the other.

The two complement each other; in fact, they work off each other. When your cardiovascular system starts becoming more invigorated as a result of all the aerobic work, your weight training will progress at a much faster tempo; conversely with the anaerobic phase of your program, your strength work, you're going to be able to run harder or bike farther or improve whatever aerobic activity you choose. So you're definitely getting mutual benefits from both these separate types of exercise.

Variety Is the Spice of Training

No matter what you do—jogging, aerobic dancing, step machines—they are all going to get pretty boring day in and day out for months at a time. But the post-pregnancy training consists of an inviting assortment of exercises. That's the beauty of it. So should there come a period of stagnation, you're free to change the program around, alter routines, even the type of stretches you do.

The diversity of my program eliminates the sheer tediousness of exercising. It enables an individual to perform at better levels on a daily basis, continually getting something new and engaging, a fresh stimulus. The upshot is that as motivation increases, the chances of burning out on a training schedule or routine decreases. Since you're challenging yourself in new ways, your body and mind are always stimulated as you learn different types of motor skills, new forms of balance and coordination.

> **With this workout you'll be pushing through the most difficult barrier of all—the barrier of boredom—and that means you're definitely going to see improvement.**

Too Much Too Soon

These are fast times. Millions of folks want instant gratification. Small wonder there is a real temptation to speed up the progress, attempting too much too soon. I think that people often get caught up in achieving goals too quickly and this can result in injury. And often this type of stress is caused by competitive factors.

I had a client whose sister ran ten miles a day; therefore, she was going to run eleven. That was her mind set. Because she was goal-oriented nothing in the world was going to stop her—except her body. She wound up in the emergency room after ripping her Achille's tendon the third day out.

When you go into the post-pregnancy training, go in with the right frame of mind, knowing that it's a long-term commitment. By doing this you're not going to set yourself up for any failures. I've discovered that if people don't achieve results as fast as they'd like (probably because their goals were totally unrealistic to begin with) they will find an excuse to cop out. Therefore my advice to you and all my other clients is to establish workable time frames that you can realistically adhere to, day to day and month to month.

Don't be tempted to slack off. The more consistent you are with your training, the more consistent you'll be with your results. In other words, the fat won't come back.

An Hour Is Just Sixty Minutes

To start realizing their fitness goals, I advise my clients to invest at least an hour a day training, three days a week. To them benefits such as peace of mind, enhanced self-esteem, boosted energy, restored health, plus looking and feeling younger are well worth the commitment. Does this mean cutting back TV by half an hour or rising thirty minutes earlier to work out? Of course it might.

Exercising is just like flossing your teeth. If you don't do a complete job, top to bottom, why bother? Just like any other health routine, such as shaving or washing your hair, the post-pregnancy training is really a necessity—not a luxury. An hour devoted to yourself is a small price to pay for health and longevity.

From the very beginning it's vital that you plan the exact time when you're going to work out, and make that a major priority in your day. Figure out your schedule at least twenty-four hours in advance because as the day drags on, it's less likely you'll find time to train. Other things just come up. You're too tired from your commute or you're simply not into it. There are hundreds of reasons to put exercising off at the last minute.

However, what I've found over the years is that successful people set up a schedule of events and then write them down. Madonna always used to do that. Every day she'd have her list of things to accomplish, neatly ordered from eight in the morning onward and naturally, right at the top of her list was workout time.

If you have flexible work hours, or if you're at home and the kids are away during a certain time, put that hour back into yourself. Schedule that special time when it's convenient for you, knowing the earlier you commit to it, the sooner you'll complete your training and the better you'll feel about yourself for the rest of the day.

> Above all else, don't give yourself latitude. If you give yourself a choice of times to exercise, you probably won't work out at all. The commitment must be firm. The time must be set.

Measure for Measure

As species we are magnificently diverse. Differences abound in our basic capabilities, particularly when it comes to our physical prowess and strength. That's why it's virtually impossible to have an absolute standard of measurement by which to judge your progress. There are simply no outside standards to go by. But there is always one single person you can measure yourself against—and that person is yourself.

Throughout this training program you will be paying close attention to the progress you make. With every workout, track how your strength has increased, how much farther you can run, or how much weight you've lost. Chart your flexibility, coordination, as well as gains in balance and your ability to concentrate. Keep those records in an orderly file. I suggest a separate workout calendar, much like the appointment calendar on your desk, to make notations and comments.

Starting Over: But Not Beginning Again

Okay, you've come back from a long business trip, had the flu, been on a vacation, or just stopped working out altogether. So what now? How do you start up again? Is there an easy way to get your commitment back on track? Read on for the good news.

At the start of your post-pregnancy training program, you naturally began at a certain level. Nonetheless, when you kick off once again, you're not going to be setting out at that same level; you'll be at a higher level.

I once had one client, a very popular actress, who suddenly quit her training sessions for over a month. After I was finally able to reach her, she confessed she didn't think working out was doing her any good. But during the conversation I convinced her to give it one more try. The next time we were together I had her perform the very same workout we did on her first day of training. I made sure she ran the same distance, lifted the same amount of weights, the same everything.

Of course she breezed right through it without even breaking a sweat; but then she wanted to do more, a lot more, because it didn't even feel like a workout to her. I said we would go back to her present level of training the next day, but as for today, I only wanted her to think about how far she had come. That's all. Suffice to say, by the very next day, she was up and raring to go.

> **Knowing where you were before as well as after is the key. That's why keeping accurate records of how far you've run or the amount of weight you've lifted is crucial. If one day you ever ask yourself why you're doing it, just perform the very first workout you ever did. You'll quickly answer the question for yourself.**

Like my client the actress, you may not pick up exactly at the level where you were, but you'll definitely get back into shape much faster than when you first started training. Be moderate the first couple of times back, see how your body responds after each training session. Don't try and get up to your previous level of fitness too soon or you might injure yourself. If you're feeling too stiff, then decrease your intensity, but continue making the daily commitment to yourself to get back into your training program.

Working Through Negative Emotions

Many times if you're down on yourself, feeling depressed, stressed out, or just plain angry, the first thing that will suffer is your training schedule, and then you'll get even more frustrated and upset. Should this happen, calm yourself and then take a moment. Remember what it feels like to begin training, all the benefits you've gotten. Recall everything you've achieved since day one. Remind yourself how much worse you'd be feeling if you never started working out. Make a list if you have to.

Throughout the post-pregnancy training, use your head as well as your heart. If you're experiencing depression, it's crucial to get out there and do something physical to relieve that frustration and stress; or if you're angry, a good way of creatively using that anger is by exerting yourself, especially running or doing weights.

> **By working out when you're feeling blue, a lot of that negative energy gets used for positive results. And that'll make you feel much better.**

What's more, your mind doesn't have to be a vacuum while training. Use the time to think through your dilemmas and worries. My clients often get a clearer picture of their personal or professional distress as they're working out. While they're breaking through physical barriers, they're breaking through mental barriers as well. I've had people create entire movie deals, restructure negotiations, even figure out how to save their marriages while training. How do I know? Because they tell me.

Water: You May Need Glasses

How many times have you been told to drink at least eight glasses of water a day? Well, I'm going to pound it into your head one more time because it's probably the most important thing you can do, especially if you're embarking on a serious exercise program. And by the way, I don't mean mere fluids like orange juice, coffee, diet sodas, or Gatorade. They contain water, but they *aren't* water.

Sixty percent of our bodies are water. Water flushes out toxins, mucus, and other organic forms of sludge. Water makes sure that waste material moves through your entire system quickly and effectively, lubricating muscles and joints on the way, plus increasing the amount of blood in our veins. This in turn helps to circulate oxygen and nutrients more efficiently, which in turn raises our energy levels.

Just like your city or town can have a water shortage, so can your body, and the symptoms may not appear as mere thirst. Depriving your body of water can induce chronic headaches, poor vision, acidic stomach, and yes, even constipation. But before you drink heartily from the tap, a word of caution. I am slightly dubious about the water quality in many parts of the country. I suggest, whenever possible, bottled springwater, low-sodium sparkling varieties, or water that's been filtered.

> **It doesn't make a difference where you begin, your body is genetically primed for fitness. All you have to do is give it a chance.**

Challenging Yourself to the Fullest

As your program evolves there're going to be certain peak periods called **plateaus**. Reaching a plateau is a magnificent testament to your fitness level. Simply stated, it occurs when you reach such great shape that your workouts have to be intensified. Let's look at your heart for example. After training for a while, it becomes so well-conditioned that now an extra half mile of running is required to reach peak aerobic level.

Plateaus are good news indeed. But they require making new assessments, establishing new fitness goals, and creating fresh areas of emphasis and interest. When you move beyond the foundation level, the choices in your training start to greatly multiply.

Take the various running techniques. After two or three weeks you might choose to do some local hill work, incorporating an incline during your workout to increase intensity. Rather than just running in the traditional way, after a month you can begin doing some different types of sidesteps and crossovers as well as stridework and sprints. I'll explain these terms later on.

Let me stress once again that progress only occurs when your muscular and cardiovascular systems are pushed to the furthest they can go. This means you have to hoist added weight, run a farther distance, or climb a little higher each time you try. But believe me, each time you surpass your previous mark, the sense of achievement will fill you with astounding pride.

My 10 Health Club Commandments

By now I suspect there may be a few of you about to join or renew a health club membership, since these are convenient places where you can work out. But even though you can shell out a hefty fee for the privilege, sometimes things turn out less than satisfactory. As the former head of a very prestigious exercise facility, I realize that some risks exist. These include the club becoming insolvent, problems with insufficiently trained staff, or equipment that's not maintained properly. Therefore, before you sign any contract, go over the following checklist.

1. First contact your local Better Business Bureau or Consumer Protection agency. Make sure that there haven't been any complaints against the club you're thinking of joining.
2. Make doubly sure by writing to the International Health, Racquet, & Sports Club Association. This is a trade association that specifically examines complaints to guarantee that clubs meet basic requirements. Their services are free. Send a self-addressed stamped envelope to them at 263 Summer Street, Boston, Massachusetts, 01120.
3. No matter how elegant or inviting the facility may appear, never join a health club prior to its opening. To be completely on the safe side, it should already have been in business for at least three years. A safer bet would be the new branch of a larger, well-established outfit.
4. Never inspect the premises during off-hour periods. This can be very deceptive. Instead, go during the peak hours of use, usually around lunch- or dinnertime. If the facility is packed with people like sardines, there's probably a severe shortage of equipment. On the other hand, should the place be practically deserted, that indicates something else may be wrong.
5. Good sanitary conditions are absolutely essential. Check the pool area, saunas, Jacuzzi, steam rooms, bathrooms, and locker rooms to make sure that they are well maintained. Don't be uptight about asking club personnel how often the water is changed, cleaned, and tested for bacteria.
6. Check to make sure that all the equipment is functioning, especially treadmills, stair climbers, and electronic bicycles. Examine

rubber surfaces for wear and tear. Investigate to see if the rubber connecting bands between flywheels are cracked or frayed.

7. While going from one area to the next, ask members what they think. What are the club's strong points? Its weak spots?

8. Make sure the majority of fitness instructors are certified, preferably by the American Council on Exercise (800-825-3636); the Aerobics and Fitness Association of America (800-445-5950); or the American College of Sports Medicine (317-637-9200).

9. Nothing is ever written in concrete. Always try to negotiate your membership fee, as well as other conditions. And never *ever* sign on the spot, no matter how hard the sales pitch. I've never heard of an offer that allegedly "expired at midnight" that wasn't available the day afterward.

10. Most important, if you should wind up having second thoughts, in almost every state you have seventy-two hours to back out and get a full refund—with no further obligation!

CHAPTER 8

Getting with the Program

There are four distinct groups of exercises that make up the post-pregnancy workout: aerobic conditioning, upper-body strength training, lower-body strength training, and abdominal routines. I've organized the program into three levels of fitness. The first is called the "Foundation Stage," which is simply the level you're at when you're a beginner.

The second phase is the "Intermediate Stage." Depending upon your present shape, you'll probably move into this category within a month or two after starting. The third is the "Advanced Stage." By this point you will be experienced enough to design a fully customized program for yourself, choosing between different exercises and challenges.

The post-pregnancy training requires three alternate days a week, such as Monday, Wednesday, and Friday. On these days you will perform the exercises in the order they are listed. If you've already been consistently working out, you may decide to start at a higher level. For instance, if you've already been using weights, then beginning at the Intermediate stage would be more appropriate.

Personalizing Your Workout

If you wish, you may split the aerobic and weight training part of your workout over different days. But should you choose this option, you must still perform one aerobic training for every strength training. The weekly total should always be three aerobic workouts and three strength workouts. You may also choose to split the strength training exercises. The exercise menus on the following pages will show how to do this. Later on there will be additional ways to personalize your exercise routine. But no matter how you break down the workouts, stretching must *always* be performed before and after each session.

Calculating Your Target Heart Rate

Before you do anything, I want you to know about one very crucial measurement. Everyone has what physiologists refer to as a **maximum heart rate**. This is the number of beats per minute that your heart is capable of during periods of peak exertion. Although every individual varies slightly, there is a general formula for determining what your maximum heart rate should be. Simply subtract your age from 220. So if you're thirty years old, then your maximum heart rate is 190. Similarly if you're fifty-five, then it would be 165.

> **Remember the formula! 220 – your age = your maximum heart rate**

However, you shouldn't be exercising at your maximum heart rate because that could pose a serious danger over a period of time, especially if you haven't been training on a regular schedule. From an aerobic point-of-view, physiologists have figured out a safe range for most individuals. This is known as your **target heart rate**.

In cardiovascular training, your target should be 70 to 85 percent of your maximum heart rate. Whether you're jogging, cycling, or rowing, this is what you should be aiming for, since it's the most efficient range for exercising.

Halfway through your aerobic training and right before the cool down, monitor your heart rate for six seconds and then multiply it by ten. This determines your heart rate per minute. There are three points where you can take your pulse. The first is the radial artery on your wrist; the second is the temporal artery which lies on the side of your forehead; and the last is the carotid artery on your neck right below your jawline.

When taking your pulse at the wrist make sure to use your second, third, and fourth fingers to feel for the pulse along the thumb side. You'll feel a definite thump when you locate it.

But no matter where you decide to take your pulse, be sure to know the location beforehand, otherwise you'll waste valuable seconds looking for it and the accuracy of the test may be affected. Compare your heart rate to those levels listed below.

Target and Maximum Heart Rate Table

Age	Maximum Heart Rate	Target Heart Rate
20	200	140 to 170
25	195	137 to 166
30	190	133 to 162
35	185	130 to 157
40	180	126 to 153
45	175	123 to 149
50	170	119 to 145
55	165	116 to 140
60	160	112 to 136
65	155	109 to 132
70	150	105 to 128

How to Reach Your Target Heart Rate

Ideally, you should perform at least twenty minutes of aerobic exercise at your target heart rate. As you start walking or running, etc., your heart rate will gradually increase, as indicated in the chart below. About one third into the activity your target heart rate should be reached. Check your pulse to make sure that you don't go above it. Then for about the last third gradually take it easier until your heart rate returns to where you started.

Aerobic Profile

```
                                  *   *   *   *   *
                           *                           *
                      *                                    *
                  *                                         *
Heart Rate:  *                                               * 60
Minutes:     0     5    10  15  20  25  30  35  40     45   50 55
```

Measuring Your Resting Heart Rate

During the post-pregnancy training it's also quite helpful to measure your resting heart rate. Go to sleep with a stopwatch next to your bed. As soon as you get up in the morning, take your pulse. Normally you should arrive at a figure of between 70 and 100 beats a minute. A number of superbly conditioned athletes have resting heart rates of as little as 50. However, while a lower resting heart rate is generally a sign of fitness, you can't be completely positive all the time.

Some men and women, even those who are quite out of shape, have remarkably low resting heart rates. What's more, your heart rate can be affected by your mood, such as when you're upset, excited, or depressed. As you initiate your program, start taking your resting heart rate once every three days. You should see the figure decreasing over time. This is a sign that your stamina is definitely improving.

But Before You Begin!

Make sure that you turn to "YOUR PERSONAL PROGRESS REPORT" at the end of this chapter. Then use this Personal Progress Report to measure your progress through the coming weeks and months. I can't begin to stress how critical this is. Because not only will you feel the improvement—you'll actually see it in black and white. And that's a tremendous motivator!

> **VERY IMPORTANT!** All the exercise groups and stretches will be detailed over the following chapters. Make sure you know beforehand how many times you should repeat each movement and the amount of weight you should be using—if any. Each exercise has been lettered for your convenience.

Level One: The Foundation Stage

To get the most out of the post-pregnancy program, a good physical foundation has to be built first. Then once you've mastered that, you can start experimenting with changing the program around to suit your style. The foundation part of my training allows you to develop practically every muscle group in your body and extend your stamina. From that point on, you can more aggressively approach the Intermediate and Advanced phases of the workout.

At this first level, I focus on overall conditioning and getting your body used to all the movements of the various exercises. Balance will also be greatly enhanced, preventing needless injuries. By strengthening the extensors and flexors of the lower legs, you allow your quadriceps and hamstring muscles to stabilize your knee. Working the calves also supports your ankles and feet. And to minimize the possibility of shin splints, I work on bettering the frontal strength of the lower legs.

During the beginning stage I take a cautious approach, because a lot of mishaps can occur at this point, especially if you've been sedentary for any period of time. My advice is to start slowly. Since you aren't competing against anyone but yourself, work at your own pace. If you try to jump ahead too fast your muscular system may not be able to handle all the types of stresses these exercises can put on your body.

While working at this first stage I advise staying with the same aerobic exercise for the duration. Then as your conditioning improves you will be able to start alternating activities.

Level One: Warm-up

Perform all the WARM-UP stretches as demonstrated in Chapter Nine: "Stretching Yourself to the Limit."

Level One: Aerobic Menu

Important: The minimum time spent on an aerobic activity should be no less than twenty minutes. In the very beginning, it is more important to get into a regular routine than to reach your target heart rate. If you are walking, start on level ground. Then over the next several weeks increase the intensity by walking faster or by walking up a grade, such as a hill.

THE 10 PERCENT RULE

As a general rule of thumb, to preclude any chance of an injury, you should only increase your workout load by no more than 10 percent each week. For example, if you're starting out with a thirty-minute walk and there's no problem, then the next week extend that to thirty-three minutes. By the end of the month you should be up to around forty minutes of walking. That's a 25 percent improvement. The same holds true for running, rowing, or any other aerobic activity. The results can be dramatic.

Note: Choose any *one* of the following and do it three times a week for at least twenty minutes. The letter and name of activity are the same as listed in Chapter Ten: "Getting to the Heart of the Matter." Be sure to write down your selection in your "Progress Report."

A) Walking, Racewalking, or Hiking
B) Jogging
C) Cycling: Stationary
D) Cycling: Outdoors
E) Swimming
F) *Low*-Impact Aerobic Dancing
H) Step-Climbing Machines

> Walking is fabulous! Especially if you've just given birth. I've virtually never heard of anyone sustaining a walking-related injury. As a matter of fact, walkers experience almost no risk of injuring muscles, ligaments, or tendons. And on top of that, walking fast actually burns more calories than running slowly— providing that you swing your arms vigorously.

Level One Strength Menu: Lower Body

Note: These exercises will appear by the same letter and name as they're shown in Chapter Eleven: "Starting Completely at the Bottom." That's why there will be "skips" in the letter order. However, you *must* perform the exercises in the order that they're given here. If you're splitting your strength training, still perform them from the top of the list on down. And once again, be certain that you write down the names of the strength exercises in your "Progress Report."

Important: You can choose either three or six days a week to work out. After every lower body, upper body, or abdominal exercise, you will see the number 1 or 2 in parentheses. This means you can decide to do *all* these exercises one after the other, or that you can split the routine. If you choose to do all the exercises, then you will work out every other day three times a week.

Alternatively, if your option is to split the routine, then you must perform those exercises numbered with (1) the first day and those numbered with (2) the very next day. This adds up to six days a week. However, no matter what your preference, you will still be doing the aerobic part of your workout only three times a week.

REPS: 25 (for each exercise)

A) The Marseille Plié (1)
G) Step-ups: Alternating (1)
I) Alternate Lunges (1)
L) Flutter Kicks (2)
N) Pelvic Thrusts (2)
U) Leg Extension (2)
V) Leg Curls (2)

General Guidelines for Weight Training

Weights will be used to enhance the results of the post-pregnancy workout. But it's imperative that you adhere to the following fundamentals of working with weights.

1. The last *3-5 reps* of every exercise should be challenging; which means you should work the muscle to the point where you really have to struggle to complete the set. As they say, you should feel the "burn."
2. If the exercise seems too easy, *increase* the weight by 2 to 5 pounds, so that you can work to guideline #1.
3. Remember to exhale as you contract the muscle and inhale as you relax the effort.
4. Consistently work the muscle group through its entire range of motion.

5. Always be in control of the movement. When using weights, lift to a 2 count and lower to a 4 count.
6. Make sure to keep a steady pace to your workout. Don't stop for any period of time unless you absolutely have to.

Level One Strength Menu: Upper Body

Important: The very first time you work out, don't use any weights. Just get familiar with the movements in each exercise. Begin using weights the *second* time you exercise. I recommend starting off with 2 to 5 pounds.

Note: These exercises will appear by the same letter and name as they're listed in Chapter Twelve: "Getting Into Top Shape." Which is why again there will be certain "skips" in the letter order.

REPS: 15 (for each exercise)

A) Power Punch (1)
B) Alternate Military Press (1)
C) Backstrokes (1)
D) Arm Circles (1)
E) Shoulder Shrugs (1)
H) Hammer Curl (1)
K) Push-ups (on Knees or Incline) (2)
L) Anterior Windmills (2)
M) Pec Push (2)
N) Tight Pec Squeeze (2)
S) Tricep Dips (2)

Level One Strength Menu: Abdomen

Note: These exercises will appear by the same letter and name as they're listed in Chapter Thirteen: "Streamlining the Stomach." And don't forget to chart your improvement on your "Progress Report."

REPS: 15 (for each exercise)

  A) Sit-ups
  B) Crunchy Crunches

Level One: Cooldown

Perform all the COOLDOWN stretches as indicated in Chapter Nine: "Stretching Yourself to the Limit."

> I always find it a good idea to carry along your workout clothes, weights, and a bottle of water with you; maybe even keep them handy in the car. You never can tell when you might have some extra time to exercise!

Level Two: The Intermediate Stage

By now you should be about a month or two into the post-pregnancy training. You've probably begun to notice significant differences in your physical condition, such as more energy and stamina, and a slimmer waistline. Now it's time to move along to the next level. At the Intermediate Stage the workout becomes more challenging and therefore more fun.

Level Two: Warm-up

Perform all the warm-up stretches as demonstrated in Chapter Nine: "Stretching Yourself to the Limit."

Level Two: Aerobic Menu

Important: To further personalize your workout, choose an additional exercise from the following list to alternate with the one that you were already performing at the Foundation Stage. If you were doing stationary cycling, for instance, incorporate that with working on a step-climbing machine.

By now you should be working out aerobically for at least 30 minutes each session. Remember the 10 percent rule and increase your time accordingly. And always remember to keep your "Progress Report" up-to-date!

NOTE: As before, all exercises will be found in Chapter Ten: "Getting to the Heart of the Matter."

A) Walking, Racewalking, or Hiking
B) Jogging, (including Intervals & Stridework)
C) Cycling: Stationary
D) Cycling: Outdoors
E) Swimming
F) High- or Low-Impact Aerobic Dancing
G) Step Classes
H) Step-Climbing Machine
I) Cross-country Skiing
J) Rowing Machine
M) Mini Trampoline

Affirm your positive attitude as you train. Practice repeating to yourself "I am committed"; "I am enthusiastic"; "I am in charge of my body"; "I am getting slimmer and stronger." Compose your own beneficial statements and as an extra motivational boost write them down on 3" x 5" file cards and then tape them near your workout area where they can be easily seen.

Level Two Strength Menu: Lower Body

Important: Once more, these exercises may be split on successive days between groups (1) and (2). Just make sure that no matter how you split them up, you perform all the exercises listed three times a week.

Note: These exercises will appear in Chapter Eleven: "Starting Completely at the Bottom."

REPS: 25 (for each exercise)

A) The Marseille Plié (1)
B) Frog Squat (1)
E) Standing Squat (1)
H) Step-ups: Single Leg (1)
J) Single-Leg Lunges (1)
K) Bench Lunges (1)
U) Leg Extension (2)
V) Leg Curls (2)
L) Flutter Kicks (2)
M) Glute Raises (2)
O) Lateral Leg Lifts (straight) (2)
P) Lateral Leg Lifts (45 Degrees) (2)
T) Inner Thigh Lift with Bench (2)
W) Basic Calf Raise (2)

CAUTION: Any time you feel faint, dizzy, nauseated, or experience muscle or joint pain or cramping of any kind, take a breather. Don't continue if the pain or condition persists. Start at a lower level of intensity next time. If the same symptoms return, consult with a physician before undertaking my training.

Level Two Strength Menu: Upper Body

Note: These exercises will appear in Chapter Twelve: "Getting into Top Shape."

REPS: 15 (for each exercise)

A) Power Punch (1)
B) Alternate Military Press (1)
C) Backstrokes (11)
F) Seated Lat Rows (1)
H) Hammer Curl (1)
I) Hammer Curl with Twist (1)

K) Push-ups (Standard) (2)
M) Pec Push (2)
P) Super Flyes (2)
R) Tricep Kickbacks (2)
S) Tricep Dips (2)

Level Two Strength Menu: Abdomen

Important: You may now also alternate abdominal exercises on different days between those numbered (1) and (2).

NOTE: These exercises will appear in Chapter Thirteen: "Streamlining the Stomach."

REPS: 20 (for each exercise)

B) Crunchy Crunches (1)
C) Alternate Elbows to Knees (1)
A) Sit-ups (2)
D) Reverse Crunch (2)
E) Power Pumps (2)

> I frown upon doing any part of your abdominal exercises in steam rooms or saunas. Even though this might seem like a great shortcut to accelerating weight loss, it actually puts a real strain on your cardiovascular and respiratory systems.

Level Two: Cooldown

Perform all the COOLDOWN stretches as indicated in Chapter Nine: "Stretching Yourself to the Limit."

> Every few weeks make sure to compare your "Progress Reports" to see how far you've come!

Level Three: The Advanced Stage

Give yourself tons of credit. You've succeeded in reaching the most difficult and most challenging part of the post-pregnancy training. From this point forward you will have the ability to fully customize your own workout. That's because you can employ any of the previous exercises or add new ones of your own.

Everything I've said so far applies to Level Three workouts as well, except that they're more intense. I've found that clients progress to the Advanced Stage without sometimes realizing it. They keep upping the training ante, looking to surmount greater and greater barriers, only to discover themselves virtually transformed. What had seemed impossible just three or four months earlier now seems like a piece of cake.

How do you know when you're ready to tackle Level Three? That's easy. The Intermediate exercises just won't satisfy you anymore. You'll literally breeze through them without thinking. Once you reach the Advanced Stage of expertise, you will start choreographing your own training routines.

Level Three: Warm Up

Perform all the WARM-UP stretches as demonstrated in Chapter Nine: "Stretching Yourself to the Limit."

Level Three: Aerobic Menu

Important: To personalize your exercise routine, you may now combine three or more of the following. Even so, still be positive that you mark your "Progress Report" every time you work out.

Note: As before, all exercises will be found in Chapter Ten: "Getting to the Heart of the Matter."

    A) Walking, Racewalking, or Hiking
    B) Jogging (Including Running Backward, Sidesteps, and Crossovers)
    C) Cycling: Stationary
    D) Cycling: Outdoors

E) Swimming
F) High- (or Low-) Impact Aerobic Dancing
G) Step Classes
H) Step-Climbing Machines
I) Cross-country Skiing
J) Rowing Machines
K) Roller-Skating (or In-line Skating)
L) Aerobic Boxing
M) Mini Trampoline
N) Jumping Rope
O) Tennis, Racquetball, Squash (and Softball, Basketball, etc.)

It rains on both optimists and pessimists. The difference is that optimists believe the skies will clear up the next day. Working out sometimes presents setbacks, but consistently maintain your optimism. You will always meet the challenge. If not today, then the next day or the day after that. Weather the frustrations of working out, and you'll always bounce back stronger and leaner than ever.

Level Three Strength Menu: Lower Body

Important: As before, you may continue splitting the exercises.

Note: These exercises will appear in Chapter Eleven: "Starting Completely at the Bottom."

REPS 25 (for each exercise)

A) The Marseille Plié (1)
C) Bent-over Tight Squat (1)
D) Bent-over Marseille Plié (1)
E) Standing Squat (1)
F) Skiing Squat (1)
H) Step-ups: Single Leg (1)
L) Flutter Kicks (1)

M) Glute Raises (1)
R) Kick Outs (1)
P) Lateral Leg Lifts (45 Degrees) (2)
Q) Lateral Leg Lifts (90 Degrees) (2)
S) Inner Thigh Lift (2)
T) Inner Thigh Lift with Bench (2)
U) Leg Extensions (2)
V) Leg Curls (2)
W) Basic Calf Raise (2)
X) Calf Raise—Heels In/Toes Out (2)
Y) Calf Raise—Toes In/Heels Out (2)

Level Three Strength Menu: Upper Body

Note: These exercises will appear in Chapter Twelve: "Getting into Top Shape."

REPS: 15 (for each exercise)

B) Alternate Military Press (1)
C) Backstrokes (1)
F) Seated Lat Rows (1)
G) Seated Rows (1)
J) Sprint Curls (1,2)
L) Anterior Windmills (1)
K) Push-ups (standard) (2)
O) Prone Bench Press (With Twist) (2)
Q) Reverse Super Flyes (2)
S) Tricep Dips (2)
T) Curls to Military Press (2)
U) Bicep Curls (2)

Level Three Strength Menu: Abdomen

Note: These exercises will appear in Chapter Thirteen: "Streamlining the Stomach."

REPS: 25 (for each exercise)

    C) Alternate Elbows to Knees (1)
    E) Power Pumps (1)
    H) Scissors (1)
    I)   Crosses (1)
    J) Dead Man's Kick (1)
    A) Sit-ups (2)
    F) Pikes (2)
    G) Alternate Pikes (2)
    B) Crunchy Crunches (2)
    D) Reverse Crunches (2)

Level Three: Cooldown

Perform all the COOLDOWN stretches as demonstrated in Chapter Nine: "Stretching Yourself to the Limit."

> One way to move through exercise barriers is by thinking about the consequences of stopping. Imagine starting to put weight on again, being less flexible and taut, as well as all the detrimental effects to your cardiovascular and nervous system. Believe me, many times the only way to move forward is by remembering exactly where you've been.

Your Personal "Progress Report"

It's extremely important when you start—as well as throughout your training—to keep accurate records of your progress. These should measure the improvements in both aerobic conditioning as well as strength areas. What follows is a basic format that you can use and tailor to your needs. You may want to photocopy these pages so that you can have an ongoing "Progress Report." Naturally, as you accelerate your training, you will have to expand your list of exercises on your "Progress Report."

Aerobic Improvement

Note: The *duration* refers to the length of time you actually walked or ran or biked, etc. *Name of activity* means walking, running, cycling, etc. *Body weight* simply means how much you weigh.

Date	Name of Activity	Duration	Body Weight
1.			
2.			
3.			
4.			
5.			
6.			
7.			
8.			

Strength Improvement: Lower Body

Note: Exercise means the name of the activity such as Alternate Lunges, Shoulder Shrugs, Sit-ups, etc. Under each date indicate the amount of weight you used and the number of repetitions performed.

Date:

_____	wt/reps	wt/reps	wt/reps	wt/reps	wt/reps	wt/reps	wt/reps
Exercise							
1.							
2.							
3.							
4.							
5.							
6.							
7.							
8.							
9.							
10.							

Strength Improvement: Upper Body

Date:

_____	wt/reps	wt/reps	wt/reps	wt/reps	wt/reps	wt/reps	wt/reps
Exercise							
1.							
2.							
3.							
4.							
5.							
6.							
7.							

Strength Improvement: Abdomen

Date:

_____	1 reps	2 reps	3 reps	4 reps	5 reps	6 reps	7 reps
Exercise							
1.							
2.							
3.							
4.							
5.							
6.							
7.							

CHAPTER 9

Stretching Yourself to the Limit

You should always perform a series of comprehensive stretches and aerobic exercises before working out. The best time to stretch is when the muscles are already warmed up and pliant. To get your muscles limber, start running in place or even around the room. Don't knock yourself out, just move at a nice, steady pace. As an alternative, do twenty-five jumping jacks, jump rope, or use a stationary bicycle. You can even dance if you want to. Just make sure that you keep active for at least five minutes. The significant thing here is to increase your blood flow and raise your muscle temperature, which in turn promotes the elasticity of muscle fibers. Avoid stretching a muscle when it's cold. You may strain yourself or cause more serious damage such as tears or ruptures in ligaments or tendons. After cooling down you must also stretch the same muscle groups. This will keep them from stiffening up and plaguing you the next day.

To promote maximum flexibility I strongly recommend *static* stretching techniques, in which you slowly extend a muscle until you experience resistance or discomfort. This process takes the muscle through its full range of movement required for working out.

While performing any stretch, breathe easily and slowly, making certain you keep breathing as you reach the limit of your extension. Avoid bouncing. Hold each stretch in the farthest position for a count of fifteen seconds. Then after relaxing for a moment, repeat it three more times.

You should stretch at least ten minutes before working out. If you've been fairly sedentary, expect to be a little stiff, but don't be concerned. I guarantee that in a few weeks you'll gradually limber up. However, if you feel any pain while stretching, stop immediately. You may be attempting too much too soon. The following warm-up isolates the muscle groups we will be concentrating on.

> I know you're anxious to start the exercises, but don't skip stretching. Warming up is an essential part of your workout routine. Because in this way your heart and circulatory system aren't suddenly taxed.

Part 1: The Warm-up

A) *Warming Up the Neck:*

1. Breathe in and lean your head over as if you were going to place your ear on your shoulder. Exhale for three seconds and bring your head back to center. Then inhale once more and bring your head to the other side and repeat the exhalation. Do each side three times.
2. With your torso held straight, inhale and twist your head to the right side. Attempt to look as far in back of you as you can. Breathe out for three seconds and bring your head forward once more. Repeat on the left. Do each side three times.

B) *Warming Up the Arms:*

1. Take a towel or handkerchief and hold it behind you, the same as if you were drying your back off after a shower. With the lower arm, pull down until you can feel the stretch in the upper arm. Hold for ten seconds. Now pull upward until you can feel the stretch in the lower arm. Hold for ten seconds. Repeat two more times on each side.
2. Grasp a chinning bar or other support (such as the top of a door) which you can hold with your feet flat on the floor. Bend your knees until your feet leave the ground. Hang still supported only by your arms for thirty seconds. Extend your feet back onto the floor and let go.

> Form is far more important than how much you can stretch. Be sure that you gradually pull yourself into a stretch. Never force your body more than it can comfortably go.

C) Warming Up the Upper Back and Shoulders:

1. Hold your arms straight out at about a forty-five degree angle to your body. Circle them forward. Make sure that your shoulders come up and down with every rotation. Do these five times and then reverse, circling your arms backward five times.
2. As if performing a shrug, pull your shoulders up as high as you can while inhaling. Hold for three seconds and then exhale, bringing them as far down as possible. Repeat five times.
3. Face a bar or the back of a chair and hold it with your hands, making sure that your feet are pointed forward and your legs are straight. Slowly crouch back and down, bending your knees in the process, until you feel the stretch in your arms and shoulders. Hold this position for thirty seconds and then straighten up.

> Now, I may not be a fashion consultant, but I do have some strong advice on what to wear while exercising. Clothes that stretch where you do are an absolute must. Above all, the fabric has to let your body breathe. And underneath everything, I recommend cotton underwear for the same reason.

D) Warming Up the Lower Back and Spine:

1. Sit on the floor with your legs straight in front of you. Grab your ankles with your hands (or as far down your legs as you can go) and pull your torso toward your knees. Make sure that your head and back are held straight and don't bounce. Hold the stretch for thirty seconds and slowly bring yourself up again.

2. Stand with your feet apart and your knees bent. Hold on to your knees with your hands. Contract the stomach and make the back arch outward as far as it can. Hold for five seconds. Inhale and push your tailbone forward, which will make the back arch inward. Hold for five seconds. Repeat four more times.

E) *Warming Up the Waist:*

1. With your feet comfortably spread apart, put the right hand on the right thigh and raise your left arm straight overhead. Start sliding the right arm down the thigh, allowing the motion to pull your body to that side. Lean over as far as you can. Let the left arm come up over your head. Don't bend the knees or allow your body to lean forward. Hold for thirty seconds and repeat on the left side.
2. Take a position with your feet well apart. Extend your arms straight out to your sides and then twist the upper body to the right side at the waist. Keep your lower body straight and rigid. Focus your eyes on your right hand as you turn as far as you can. Hold for three seconds and then come around to the left side. Now focus on your left hand for three seconds. Perform each side five more times.
3. Stand straight with feet apart and your arms outstretched in either direction. Now imagine that there are two walls on either side about six inches out of reach. Keeping the hips still and the shoulders level, pretend that you are bending over to try and touch the wall on the right side with your fingertips. Hold for five seconds. Now do the same thing on the left. Repeat three times on both sides.

When performing your stretching routines, wood floors or tightly carpeted surfaces are far superior to tile or concrete.

F) *Warming Up the Thighs:*

1. Standing next to a wall and, supporting yourself with your right hand, use your left hand to take hold of your right foot. Pull your heel up toward your buttocks. Make sure to keep your body straight and erect. Hold this for twenty seconds. Now face the opposite direction, your left hand on the wall, and grasp your left foot with your right hand. Repeat.
2. Bend your knees and balance yourself by placing your fingers on the floor. Extend one leg straight back as far as it will go. The other leg should stay bent with the knee over the ankle. Imagine that someone is pressing down on your buttocks, pushing your groin toward the ground. Lean into the position and hold for thirty seconds. Repeat with the opposite leg.

> **Make sure to keep on giving every muscle group a good stretch. "Cold" muscles are much more prone to injury.**

G) *Warming Up the Calves:*

1. Stand about three feet away from a wall. In order to properly stretch the upper calf muscle put both your hands on the wall at shoulder height and lean forward. Keep the left foot stationary and step forward with the right foot until your toes are about six inches from the wall. Now bend your right knee as far as you can and push down with your left heel. Make sure your left leg is held straight and that both feet are pointed forward. Hold for thirty seconds. Now reverse sides.
2. In the same manner as the previous exercise, stand three feet away from the wall and place your hands against it at shoulder height. Keep the left leg in place and step forward with the right foot, until your toes are about six inches from the wall. However, this time bend the left knee and keep the right leg straight. Feel the stretch in the lower calf. Hold for thirty seconds. Then reverse sides.

H) Warming Up the Achilles Tendon:

1. Put your hands on the floor and extend your legs in back of you. Balance yourself on your hands and on the balls of your feet and your toes. Your stomach and legs are off the ground. Press down on your right heel as far as you can go toward the floor. Feel the stretch in the back of the leg and hold for five seconds. Now relax that leg and press down with the left heel. Hold for five seconds. Do each side four more times.

I) Warming Up the Hamstrings:

1. Sit spread legged on the floor and twist your body so that you're facing the right leg. Grab your right ankle (or as far down your leg as you can) with your hands and pull your torso forward. Make sure to keep your back and head straight. Hold for thirty seconds. Now reverse and repeat on the right side.
2. From a standing position, with legs about an inch apart, bend over at the waist and hang down. Now reach your arms behind you and clasp them together behind your knees. Pull your chest toward your knees and hold for thirty seconds. Make sure that your legs remain straight and that your knees are firm. Relax and slowly straighten up, one vertebra at a time.

When warming up the hamstrings, it's vital that you don't bounce or strain yourself. In fact, you should never bounce or strain yourself while stretching any muscle.

J) Warming Up the Groin:

1. While sitting on the floor, bend your legs inward so that the souls of your feet touch each other. Grab your ankles and pull your body forward. Push your knees down with your elbows in the process. Then see if your forehead can reach your feet. Hold for thirty seconds and slowly sit up, one vertebra at a time.

2. Stand with your feet as wide apart as you comfortably can. Bend forward keeping the soles flat on the floor. Allow the palms of your hands to touch the floor in front of you. (If you can't bend all the way down, then hold on to a chair or other support). Bend your right knee, making sure to keep the left leg straight. Feel the stretch in your inner left thigh and groin. Hold for ten seconds. Now bring yourself up and bend the left knee the exact same way. Hold for ten seconds. Repeat twice more on either side.

K) Warming Up the Buttocks:

1. Get down on your hands and knees. Move your left leg back so that the left knee is even with your right foot. Lower your chest toward the right knee. To increase the stretch, try pushing out your left leg behind you even more. Hold for thirty seconds. Repeat using the opposite leg.

By the way, I always tell my clients never to exercise on an empty stomach. If you haven't eaten for over two hours, make sure to have a light snack and a glass of water at least twenty to thirty minutes before doing your initial stretching.

Part 2. The Cooldown

As I've mentioned, stretching after the post-pregnancy workout is a very critical factor in achieving the results you want. All the stretches you did for the warm-up can also be utilized during the cooldown period. But to help break the monotony, I have included some additional stretches as well. These can also be used during the warm-up period. The choice is yours. Where there is no appropriate alternative, do the warm-up stretch.

Never skip cooling down. These stretches are absolutely crucial for avoiding any serious injury. And because cooling down further makes your muscle groups pliable and strong, it's a vital step toward reaching that slim, glorious body!

A) Cooling Down the Neck:

Do warm-up stretches.

B) Cooling Down the Arms:

Do warm-up stretches.

C) Cooling Down the Upper Back and Shoulders:

1. First hold your right arm in front of you. Then bend it and hold your left shoulder with your right hand. Take your left arm and grab your right elbow. Pull your right elbow toward you for five seconds. Relax and do three more times. Then grab your right shoulder with your left and repeat the process.
2. Go down on all fours. Bring the right knee as close to your nose as possible by arching your back upward. Then stretch the leg back and up while at the same time raising your head. The arch of your back should now be pointed downward. Also make certain that your arms don't bend. Perform four more times and then repeat with the left leg.

D) Cooling Down the Lower Back and Spine:

1. Sit on the floor with your legs straight in front of you and your hands on the floor in back. Raise your left leg and bend it over the right. Place the left foot to the right of the right knee. Now bring your left arm under your left leg and grab your right thigh. Keeping your head and back straight, slowly twist your torso to the right side and hold, using your right arm for support. Hold for thirty seconds and repeat to the left side.

or

2. Lie facedown on the mat with your body straight. Bring your hands to the center of your chest. Turn them inward so that the middle fingers touch each other. Check that your palms are flat on the floor. Slowly raise your torso by extending your arms, much like a push-up. Hold that position for ten seconds. Then gradually twist your body to the right, turning your head to look over your right shoulder. Make sure that toes are on the floor and your back straight. Hold for twenty seconds. Slowly turn back and face downward. Hold for ten seconds. Then repeat the movement on the opposite side, looking over your left shoulder.

or

3. (*Note:* This is a more advanced stretch) Lie on your back with your arms at your sides with your hands on the floor, palms down. Bending only at the waist, bring your legs straight up, using your hands as support. Continue the motion until you touch your toes behind your head. Increase the stretch by placing your knees behind your head. If your feet don't touch the floor in back of you, bring them down as far as you can. Don't force yourself. Hold the maximum position for thirty seconds and then, using only your abdominal muscles, raise your legs straight over your head and down to the starting position.

E) *Cooling Down the Waist:*

Do warm-up stretches.

F) *Cooling Down the Thighs:*

1. Lie on your back with your legs straight out. Bend your right knee and grab the leg with both hands. Now extend the leg upward, holding it with your hands behind the thigh and the ankle. Pull it toward your chest and hold for twenty seconds. Now repeat with the left leg.

G) *Cooling Down the Calves:*

Do warm-up stretches.

H) Cooling Down the Achilles Tendon:

1. Stand on a book, a box, or a stair step using the toes and balls of the feet. Allow your heels and insteps to stay free in the air. Using the right foot for balance, push down on your left heel until you feel the stretch. Hold five seconds and repeat three times. Now reverse and stretch on the right side.

> When exercising down on the floor, always get up slowly. This helps to avoid dizziness and weakness in the legs.

I) Cooling Down the Hamstrings:

1. Sit on the floor with both legs straight in front of you, knees close together. Lift the right leg and put the right heel on the toes on the left foot. Extend your arms in front of you and try and touch the toes of your right foot. Keep your back and head straight. Bend over as far as you can go and hold for thirty seconds. Now reverse, putting the left heel atop the right toes.

J) Cooling Down the Groin:

1. Sit on the floor with your legs as wide apart as possible. Place your hands on the floor in front of you. Start bending over. See how far you can lean between your legs by letting your fingers creep forward. Feel the stretch in the front of the groin and hold for thirty seconds. Slowly relax and sit up.

K) Cooling Down the Buttocks:

1. Kneel back with your butt resting on your ankles. Place your hands in back of you for support on either side, fingers facing forward. Now arch your back upward, so that the buttocks come off the knees. Your abdomen should be pushing toward the ceiling as well. Hold the stretch for ten seconds and then repeat four more times.

Just try to clear your mind. Continue focusing on the moves. This will not only increase body awareness, but relieve any leftover stress you may still have.

L) Cooling Down the Whole Body:

1. Lie flat on your back with your feet out straight. Now raise your knees up. Keeping both shoulders on the ground, drop your knees to your right side and hold for thirty seconds. At the same time, turn your head so that it is facing left. If you can, extend this stretch by taking your left foot (which should be on top) and straightening it out, so that the toes are touching the ground. Slowly bring your knees up and drop them to your left side and repeat, with your head turning right.

2. Right after the stretch above, let your knees come back down with your legs straight out. Reach your arms over your head. Imagine that ropes are attached to your arms and legs and you are being stretched in between them. Hold for ten seconds. Relax and then repeat two times. Lie still for at least another thirty seconds.

3. Slowly get up on your feet, keeping your knees bent and head hanging over. Roll your torso up slowly, one vertebra at a time, until you are standing up straight, legs apart. Now inhale as you raise your arms upward over your head. Exhale and let them down again. Repeat this for three deep breaths. If you like, as you inhale, you may rise up on your toes.

CHAPTER 10

Getting to the Heart of the Matter

Exercises that demand large amounts of oxygen over extended periods of time are called aerobic. Aerobic exercises compel the body to improve those systems responsible for the transportation of oxygen. Through proper aerobic conditioning your lung capacity not only expands, but the heart becomes more proficient with every beat, since the main heart chamber actually enlarges in size.

All aerobic exercises use Long Slow Distance (LSD) as the primary method of building endurance. Even though LSD training first appears to refer to jogging, it actually comprises a much wider range of activities, all of which share one characteristic: the ability to accelerate your heart rate up to 70 to 85 percent of its maximum capacity for at least twenty to forty minutes.

Make sure to take additional calcium, particularly if you're breastfeeding. This helps replenish your bones and makes them more resilient to the strains of various aerobic activities.

Aerobic Exercise	Calories Burned (per hour)
Aerobic Boxing	790
Aerobic Dancing	820
Basketball	550
Bicycling 6 mph	245
Bicycling 10 mph	350
Bicycling 14 mph	460
Cross-country Skiing	730
Jogging 5 mph	720*
Jogging 7 mph	935*
Jumping Rope	760
Racquetball or Squash	550
Rollerskating	425
Running in Place	675
Rowing	465
Stationary Bicycling	**
Step Classes	825
Step-Climbing Machines	***
Swimming 30 yds/min	325
Swimming 50 yds/min	550
Tennis (Singles)	420
Trampoline	405
Walking 2 mph (Level Ground)	250
Walking 3 mph "	340
Walking 5 mph "	490

NOTE: Many of these figures can be affected by intensity, resistance, rate of incline, or the use of weights.

*Most treadmills in gyms will now give you a calorie count.
**Use same figures as bicycling but deduct 60 calories.
***These are usually high tech. It's best to check the readout.

The Pros and Cons of Aerobic Exercises

No one aerobic exercise is perfect for everyone. While walking might be a wonderful idea, especially in a spectacularly scenic area such as Boulder, Colorado, you might think twice about it if you lived in a big metropolis. Similarly, southern Californians may have more time out of the year to use their pools than residents of Maine.

But unless you truly have a passion for any one exercise, I usually find that people become bored after a period of time. That's why I insist on alternating aerobic activities rather than focusing on just one. Even though all of them raise the heart rate, there are differences, particularly in how challenging they are.

A stationary bicycle may fit easily into your basement, but a mountain bike will give you a far more vigorous and exciting workout. I'm also a big believer in backpacking and hiking. Along the way you might even decide to take up rock or mountain climbing.

Aerobic exercise can be the most fun and stimulating part of your training. So don't get into an aerobic rut. Vary your routine.

A) Walking, Racewalking, or Hiking

Pros: The easiest of all aerobic exercises is no doubt one of the best, especially if you're somewhat out-of-shape to begin with. Walking only fifteen miles a week, three miles a day over five days, will consume between 1,100 and 1,600 calories depending on how fast you walk, what you weigh, as well as where you walk. To increase the intensity swing the arms emphatically or pump weights as you walk.

But the easiest way to maximize results is by walking uphill. For instance, if you burn 400 calories walking at 4 mph on level ground, then you can increase that to 550 calories on a 5 percent grade. A 10 percent grade will take up to 760 calories, and a 20 percent grade will take you over 1,000 calories an hour. Small wonder climbing stairs is so exhausting. That's a 50 percent grade right there.

Unlike running or jogging or other high impact aerobic activities, walking poses virtually no threat to ligaments, tendons, muscles, and joints. Walkers are unlikely to be plagued by tendonitis, sprains, strains, or stress fractures. Always remember to walk heel-toe while keeping your arms moving back and forth. If convenient, you can walk around a track, on a treadmill, or take an inspiring hike through local hills or mountains.

For post-pregnancy training I recommend walking between 3 and 5 mph when you're on level ground. Take your pulse every ten minutes to make sure that you are reaching your target heart rate. As your aerobic condition improves and your heart rate plateaus, you will have to work harder by walking faster. Above 5 mph you will be racewalking, which calls for swinging your arms even more fervently. If this doesn't appeal to you, simply find steeper hills or use hand or ankle weights—or both.

Cons: Boredom is one of the complaints I often hear about, especially if you don't live near a park, a reservoir, or some other place where you can freely enjoy the scenery. Weather may also be a factor, as well as the longer period of time it usually takes to get a good workout this way. Nevertheless, the major drawback is that many people simply don't walk fast enough. To make sure that you're going at the right pace, a good rule of thumb is to count the steps that you take per minute.

To go an average of 2 mph you must take about 65 steps a minute; likewise, 3 mph requires 100 steps a minute; 4 mph needs 135 steps, and 5 mph uses about 170 steps.

> **Whether you're jogging or walking, make sure that the surface beneath your legs is level. Try to steer away from hard-surfaced roads or paved sidewalks, for these can be murder on your feet. My personal preference is soft running tracks or grassy trails.**

B) Jogging

Pros: You don't have to be a marathoner to reap the benefits of running. In fact, jogging for about thirty minutes four times a week will probably give you most of the aerobic benefits you want. But a lot of people aren't up to running the whole time when they first begin, so I recommend starting with a walking and jogging program.

Say you aerobically exercise for twenty-five minutes. The first week take 20 percent of that time (or five minutes) and devote it to jogging. The other twenty minutes you'll be walking. By the second week increase your time to thirty minutes but keep the ratios the same.

The third week keep the time the same but see if you can raise it to twelve minutes of jogging and eighteen minutes of walking per thirty-minute period. Gradually increase the ratio of jogging to walking until by the fifth week you're jogging and walking the same amount of time. After nine weeks make your target 90 percent jogging to 10 percent walking over thirty-five minutes.

Cons: Muscle pulls, damage to the bones, joints, tendons, and ligaments are the primary reasons not to jog. Inadequate footwear can contribute to hurting yourself, so make sure that your jogging shoes have enough support and cushioning to insulate your feet from the constant pounding.

Jogging on a rubber treadmill will decrease the impact, and hence the incidence of injuries, but it may also increase the boredom, even if the treadmill does feature different speeds and inclines. And unless you live in a town like San Diego where the climate is moderate all year round, there may be some days when you're tempted to forego your outdoor workout, especially when the temperature goes over 90 degrees or sinks below 20.

When it comes to exercise shoes, no matter what the aerobic activity, always wear one a little wider than you're accustomed to with good absorption. This will help to minimize the chance of stress fractures.

INTERMEDIATE AND ADVANCED RUNNING TECHNIQUES

1. **Intervals:** Let's say you're planning to run for forty minutes. For the first ten minutes just warm up—a nice easy jog to prepare your body for a little more strenuous pace. Then the next ten minutes pick up speed. For twenty to thirty minutes do a section of intervals, which means a number of thirty-second sprints that

bring your maximum heart rate up to 80 to 90 percent of capacity, followed by an easy pace to recover. After each sprint allow yourself a minute for this, and then sprint again.

For more aggressive training, increase the intensity of the interval. Instead of thirty seconds, sprint for one minute long. But remember: no matter what the duration of the sprint, whether it's thirty seconds or a minute, the recovery section should be twice as long. In other words if you've sprinted for a minute, then give yourself a full two-minute recovery at the slower pace, 60 to 75 percent of your maximum heart rate.

2. **Stridework:** During your road work you'll be picking out certain landmarks. While running toward them, increase the length of your stride. This will make you cover more ground in less time. Think of stridework as if you were taking giant steps during jogging. Again, do this a series of times just like the intervals described above. Stridework will also bring your maximum heart rate up to 80 to 90 percent of maximum capacity.

> My advice is that you should never run outdoors during very hot or humid weather. Heat can place a tremendous strain on the body's basic systems. Don't risk it!

3. **Running Backward:** Running backward, especially uphill, helps build more coordination and more agility. It also strengthens the calves as well as puts a little more pressure on the frontal thighs. But be sure that you know where you're going. Check out your path for any obstacles or cracks.

4. **Sidesteps:** For maximum results, sidestepping is also done while going uphill. On the balls of your feet simply move sideways, right to left, left to right, or in both directions.

5. **Crossovers:** Moving to the right, first cross your left foot in front of your right. Next bring your right forward and parallel with your left. Then cross your left foot in back of your right and finally step back with your right, so that once again it's parallel with your left. Start all over again. To move to the left reverse the movement, this time with your right foot crossing over your left and then in back.

Try combining sidesteps, crossovers, and running backward while running up hills. If you have a running partner, another variation would be follow the leader, where one person would initiate different patterns of short intensity, maybe only over ten to twenty yards, whereupon the other person exactly imitates his or her partner. The key here is extremely quick movements and fast reaction times. Follow the leader is great training for more athletic competitions such as sports involving lateral and horizontal agility.

Since a lot of the primary muscle groups are involved in these exercises, they can sometimes get extremely tight. Therefore special emphasis should be placed on stretching the hamstrings, hip flexors, quadriceps, low back, and glutes.

A WORD ABOUT RUNNING SHOES

You should rotate your shoes. Have at least two pairs of running shoes and constantly rotate them so that each shoe always has a good sole on it. Your shoes should also have excellent support, good stability, plus the proper foot alignment. Some people lean to the inside or outside of their heel when they run. When your heel hits the grounds it's called a heel strike. If you have a podiatrist or other sports physician, bring him or her a pair of your old running shoes or sneakers in order to find out what type of heel strike you have. From that they can recommend the type of running shoes best suited to your stride. Here are some other rules:

- Jog on the gentlest, most level surface you can find. Grass and soil are ideal since they help absorb some of your foot's impact. Concrete or other hard surfaces post the greatest risk. I don't recommend running on the beach. Sand can cause your legs to twist and strain.
- Always be certain you land on your heels. Allow the downward movement to smoothly take you forward but remember to always push off with your toes. Never run flat-footed.

- Don't run like a duck with you toes pointing out right and left. Jog by placing one foot in front of the other in line with the center of your body. Toes should be facing straight ahead.
- Keep your feet close to the ground.
- Knees must be brought forward with every stride. Check to see that your heel lands right underneath your knee. If it doesn't, your strides are too long. Make them shorter.
- Always make certain that you lean forward a bit.
- Be sure that your arms are bent at a 90-degree angle. Don't make a fist or clench your hands tightly. Keep the fingers loose.
- Arm movement equates to speed. The more energetically you use your arms, the faster you will be traveling.

If you're exercising a lot outdoors, especially in urban areas, make sure to take extra amounts of antioxidants, particularly betacarotene and vitamins C and E. These all help combat the effects of prolonged exposure to auto emissions, air pollution, pesticides, as well as other toxins that may be around.

C) Cycling: Stationary

Pros: The major advantage of stationary cycling is that it's safe and convenient. You can do it indoors listening to music, while reading or even watching television. It's extremely user friendly, especially for older folks who may have bone or joint problems. From an aerobic point of view, speeds of less than 10 miles per hour have little value. I recommend a minimum speed of 16 miles per hour to receive the right aerobic benefits.

A stationary bicycle should have instrumentation to calculate speed and distance. The more advanced models should show how many rpms you're working at, plus they have an ergometer, a device that reveals how many calories you're expending on an hourly basis.

Nonetheless, the key is setting the resistance mechanism properly, to a point where you'll be working at your target heart rate. The resistance should always stay consistent over the full distance you're pedaling.

Besides stationary bicycles there are always the new electronic ones, such as Lifecycles, which can vary the intensity of the experience to simulate outdoor biking. These devices might be somewhat more challenging.

Cons: Boredom is actually the least of the difficulties with stationary cycling. The major problem is that no matter how you slice it, biking inside is just not the same as biking outside, primarily because it just takes a lot more effort to reap the results. When cycling outdoors, not only are you overcoming the wind and atmospheric resistance, but you're actually expending energy in propelling your body forward.

To compensate on a stationary cycle, resistance must be increased. But from doing this your legs may become too fatigued to keep up the speed, in which case you slow down and lose aerobic benefits. So even though stationary bikes are popular, I'm not their greatest fan.

D) Cycling: Outdoors

Pros: This exercise is one of my favorites. With the rising popularity of the "mountain" bike, that hybrid vehicle with wide tires, deep treads, spread-out handlebars, and an elaborate gear system, once difficult terrain has become easy to conquer. Although mountain bikes are built tough, they're stable to ride, delivering far more solid support than conventional "racing" bikes, which can be knocked out of alignment by a bad bump.

With as many as eighteen gears, mountain bikes can definitely alleviate the boredom so prevalent with other kinds of aerobic exercise, as you plan out a new travel itinerary each time you ride. To get the aerobic benefits of outdoor riding you must bike at least five miles in twenty minutes—or 15 mph on relatively level ground. I recommend cycling at least three times each week. But first see how far you can go the first day without becoming overly fatigued. From then on increase your mileage by 10 percent a week.

Cons: If you don't have access to a park or rural surroundings, biking through urban traffic can be a nightmare, often creating more stress than it relieves. Like any moving vehicle, there's always a threat of accident or collision. To offset any possible head injuries I suggest wearing a helmet at all times when you're biking. Here are some additional pointers:

- Make certain that your seat is set at the right height. If not you can get serious knee and ankle strain. While sitting make sure that the ball of your foot can extend almost fully to the pedal on the down-stroke.
- Don't tense your arms or shoulders. Neither should you grip the handlebars too tightly. Relax and stay loose as you ride.
- Stay in a lower gear whenever possible. Pedaling in a higher gear may offer you greater resistance, but it might also have detrimental effects upon your knees. Doing spurts in higher gears for short distances is perfectly acceptable. However, consistency of speed is what's truly important here.
- Try utilizing toe clips. They look like a metal stirrup attached to the pedal in which you insert your foot. By forcing your leg to work on the way up as well as down, stirrups increase the efficiency of cycling by about 30 percent.

CYCLING AND RUNNING: HAPPY TOGETHER

Variety is the spice of training life. Which is why running and cycling can be alternated or combined. The duration of the bike ride must be 50 percent greater than your running time to achieve equivalent results. The reason cycling should be longer is that when you're riding a bike there's lots of gliding involved, especially when going downhill, so you don't always have to work.

> Running constantly requires an individual to push against the forces of gravity. There's no gear box to soften the job up; hence it's the more concentrated exercise.

E) Swimming

Pros: Water has some very intriguing qualities besides being refreshing and cool. Because water offsets up to 75 percent of a person's body weight, it's the perfect environment for people with weight problems, arthritis, or various physical impairments, who might otherwise injure themselves performing aerobic activities on dry land. Swimming works practically every muscle group in your body, while the water's natural buoyancy serves to cushion any excessive pressure upon joints and bones. No wonder it's the exercise of choice for pregnant women.

Continuous swimming is naturally the best approach, even better if you can go for thirty minutes straight. However, few beginners are in this type of peak condition. If you're just starting out, I advocate swimming a few laps at first and then resting. Then in successive weeks make the rest periods shorter and shorter (use a waterproof watch if you have to), until you can go half an hour nonstop.

Cons: Unfortunately, while swimming is one of the best ways to stay in condition, from a fat-burning point-of-view it has a minimal effect. This is because the core temperature of the muscle groups don't heat up as much, plus the fact that you get an exceptional amount of glide while you're in the pool. The bottom line is that even though you're going to burn calories, you're not apt to burn great amounts of fat, as in land-based exercises.

While owning your own pool is ideal, since you can control what goes in and out of it, most of us rely on gyms or health clubs. And therein lies the problem. These pools are not only saturated with chlorine, they're often saturated with bacteria, some of which can lead to stinging eyes and discolored hair, while others to ear and sinus infections.

While most health facilities are bound by state laws to enforce stringent codes, you and I know this is sometimes not the case. Therefore, before joining any health club, check to make sure the pool area is being tended properly. Finally, swimming in oceans and lakes can also pose problems, particularly if there's pollution or sewage contamination, so be cautious there as well. Here are some additional pointers:

- While you're immersed in the water, your heart slows down by fifteen beats a minute, because swimming allows your circulatory system to function more efficiently. In order to compensate aerobically you must then decrease your target heart rate accordingly. To calculate your new maximum heart rate within the water, men should subtract half their age from 195 and women their full age from 205. As before, your target heart rate is now 70 to 85 percent of this number.
- The stroke I encourage for optimal results is the forward crawl, also known as freestyle swimming. Although the sidestroke and the

breaststroke are less intense, they can be substituted from time to time, as can the butterfly and the backstroke.

- It's better to perform slow and sweeping motions rather than a bunch of fast moves, which tend to fight the water instead of flowing with it.
- To minimize harm to your hair, try rubbing in a few drops of baby or mineral oil before you enter the pool. Always put on a bathing cap and make sure to shampoo thoroughly after you get out.
- Snug goggles are a big plus for defending your eyes against the ravages of chlorine. However, if your eyes are bleary and red even after wearing them, then the PH balance of the pool may need serious adjustment. Talk to the person in charge.

F) High- or Low-Impact Aerobic Dancing

Pros: Participating in a fun class gives a lot of people the extra boost they need to complete an aerobic workout. There's a special bond that seems to form between those who have been attending the same class for a period of time, and this can also make the activity much more enjoyable. Even for those who are gym-shy, there are many books and videotapes which make it easy to perform these exercises at home.

However, aerobic dancing is only effective if you're working at your target heart rate. Check your pulse every five minutes to make sure. Aerobics also improves grace and dexterity and adds bounce to your step. Be positive beforehand that any class you take features stretching, a warm-up period, at least twenty minutes of aerobic exercise, and a sufficient cooldown of at least ten minutes.

Cons: The enthusiasm for high-impact aerobic dancing is somewhat tarnished, mostly because of the high incidence of torn ligaments, knee sprains, shin splints, and bruised hips. This should come as no surprise to anyone acquainted with the laws of physics. When jumping up and down, you literally land with the impact of three times your weight, which really does a number on your skeletal system.

In any event, what I suggest to many of my clients is low-impact aerobics. While this lacks some of the glamour of the high-impact variety, it's a lot safer in the long run. The focus in low-impact aerobics is on keeping one foot on the ground at all times, which minimizes the risk of injury. Consequently, wild jumping jacks are out and marching with exaggerated arm movement is in. Here are some further pointers:

- It's absolutely imperative to examine the floor. Nothing can damage your joints and muscles faster than a floor which doesn't help absorb your body's impact. Don't even think about exercising on a cement floor, or a cement floor that has been covered over with carpet. Either one will be murder on your legs. Without a doubt the most superior surface is hardwood, but it should always be cushioned underneath with a layer of sponge or an air space.
- Don't give up after the first class. Aerobic dancing is as much about coordinating your brain as your feet. Instructors all rely on individual routines, and it might take a couple of lessons for you to get the hang of it. If you're tripping over your feet, don't worry about it. All the people in the front row were also klutzes when they first came in.
- Don't be embarrassed to make inquiries about the instructor's qualifications before enrolling in any exercise class. As with any other professional, they should have the proper training and credentials.

My advice is to avoid those situations where the instructor seems more concerned with "putting on a show" rather than relating to the needs of those taking the class.

G) Step Classes

Pros: These have become very popular of late. Doing step has basically all the great benefits of low-impact aerobics. It works the calves and thighs especially hard, which is great for developing tone and muscles in those areas. Because one, two, or even three steps can be used, the intensity of the exercise can be controlled, a big plus as you plateau.

The majority of women need only one step to get great results. However, if you've got long legs, you may want to use two. Three steps should only be used at the most advanced level—if ever.

Cons: Step classes incorporate many of the same leg and hand movements as aerobic dance, but require greater agility. The process of stepping up and down can be quite disorienting at first, and because of this, the initial injury rate is somewhat higher. These injuries can also be of a more serious nature, since falling or tripping from a raised platform can produce greater trauma than if you're on level ground. Also avoid being competitive. That's when people most frequently get hurt.

- During any step class, you must be certain that you're landing on the entire foot, not just the toes or the heel.
- If you can't coordinate your arms and legs, focus on your footwork. This will help you from tripping up or taking a spill.

H) Step-Climbing Machines

Pros: These devices give you a great lower-body workout. They have practically all the aerobic benefits of step classes, but are virtually injury-free since there's no impact or moving around involved. Reading or watching television is also a possibility with this exercise. Step-climbing machines generally measure the hourly amount of calories you're burning, plus they have resistance controls, which is an excellent way to keep your workout challenging.

Cons: Like treadmills or cycles, these devices really don't give you much of an upper body workout. In this respect they are somewhat inferior to good step classes which usually include enthusiastic arm movements. Another drawback for step-climbing machines, as with other repetitive aerobic devices, is the boredom. For this reason step climbing should always be augmented with exercise classes or outdoor activities.

I) Cross-country Skiing

Pros: There's no doubt about it. This is one of the top aerobic exercises—if not the best—for improving stamina. Cross-country skiing involves every major muscle group, not just the ones in the legs. Thus, in many ways it's superior to either jogging or cycling. Because this exercise is done at fairly high altitudes and in cold temperatures, it adds rigor to the workout as your body is further challenged by the environment. When you cross-country ski, heavier clothing is required and this added weight further contributes to the effectiveness of the exercise.

Cons: The greatest advantage of cross-country skiing is also its biggest disadvantage. You have to be around snow. Fortunately there are numerous machines which simulate the process of cross-country skiing, including the popular NordicTrack. Unlike conventional exercise bikes or treadmills, these machines provide a far more comprehensive workout. But like other machines they can become boring.

J) Rowing Machines

Pros: Only the cross-country ski machines give a better overall workout than these. Rowing machines empower the upper and lower body as well as strengthen the abdominal muscles. It's an efficient exercise in which aerobic results can be attained in a minimal amount of time. Usually they're easy to store and convenient to use.

Cons: Let's face it. Rowing can get pretty boring. But that's not the major complaint against these machines. A lot of people claim that rowing simply hurts their backs. This isn't surprising, because maintaining proper form on a rowing machine requires patience and is fairly difficult to master.

Often beginners put their backs into it—which is exactly the wrong thing to do. Your back should stay straight but basically uninvolved in the total movement. The only body parts that should be working are your legs, shoulders, and arms. Keeping your stomach muscles tight also helps.

> Shortness of breath is a sure sign you should slow down during any aerobic exercise. Immediately ease up on what you're doing. Work at your own comfortable rhythm until you can breathe easily again.

K) Roller Skating (or In-line Skating)

Pros: Recent studies have demonstrated that roller skating at 10 mph is equal, from an aerobic point-of-view, to jogging at 5 mph. However, this is only valid if you're skating continuously over the same period of time.

If you're tempted to just coast along, which often occurs in roller-skating or outdoor cycling, then the results will be less beneficial.

Cons: Unlike cycling, this is not an exercise readily picked up by adults, even those who were real terrors on skates in their childhoods. The most common problem with roller-skating, and especially in-line skating on a single set of linear wheels, are ankle injuries and fatigue. Skates are harder to stop than a bicycle, so collisions and pratfalls are a greater nuisance. I strongly recommend helmets, wrist guards, and kneepads while skating to escape serious damage.

Note: While ice-skating appears to be in a similar category, I'm afraid it's not. There's just too much glide in ice-skating to make it a consistent aerobic workout. The only exception is if you're training for figure or speed skating. Otherwise, leisurely going around the rink just doesn't make it.

L) Aerobic Boxing

Pros: Self-defense is obviously an invaluable skill to develop. Today there are classes in boxing for both men and women, and they have my strong support as a comprehensive workout, both upper and lower body. To build up stamina you jump rope or jog or both for a substantial period of time. Hand and eye coordination are developed, as well as precise rhythm, after working out on the punching bag. Usually aerobic boxing is more consistent than other stop-and-go sports since you are constantly training, constantly in motion.

Cons: There is some possibility of injury here, particularly if you're wearing gloves that don't fit or aren't padded properly. Some women may feel uncomfortable squaring off against others, but in most classes if you don't want to fight anyone else you certainly don't have to. The training is the key, not the sparring. Lastly, aerobic boxing classes may be more difficult to locate.

> Besides its aerobic benefits, aerobic boxing may be the best way to work out aggression, particularly if you imagine the punching bag as your boss's face.

M) Mini Trampoline

Pros: Rebounding on the mini trampoline often reduces the risk of injury because its elastic surface absorbs much of the impact. And while it requires no more room than a stationary bicycle or a rowing machine, it's usually easier to store. The square or rectangular variety are generally more stable than the round models. The mini trampoline is a minimally adequate replacement for exercises such as jogging and aerobics, which tend to have greater impact on the joints and tendons.

Cons: Unfortunately, the surface absorbs much of the benefits as well. Studies have consistently proven that jumping on the trampoline burns up even less calories than running in place for the same amount of time.

By decreasing the load of gravity and giving you that extra bounce, it actually reduces the amount of work your body has to perform. In other words, the muscles in your legs get shortchanged because the trampoline simply springs you into the air.

N) Jumping Rope

Pros: George Foreman does it—need I say more? Jumping rope is a supremely beneficial aerobic exercise, and I can't recommend it highly enough. Instead of spending hundreds or even thousands of dollars for a stationary bicycle or cross-country machine, you can purchase this item for about fifteen bucks. And here I'm talking about a first-class rope with all the trimmings, including plastic links and foam rubber handles. Jumping rope forces you to focus on what you're doing, improving your agility, stamina, and sense of balance in the process.

In terms of pure efficiency, perhaps no other exercise can raise your heart rate as quickly as jumping rope. Take my word for it. Twenty minutes of continuous rope jumping is a major aerobic achievement.

Cons: For the uninitiated, jumping rope is tough. It requires hand-eye coordination skills as well as excellent muscular endurance. Because it requires so much energy so soon, those who aren't already in great aerobic shape may find jumping rope more frustrating than cycling or even cross-country machines. Also it may be somewhat unnerving to see a five-year-old girl doing it when you can't. Some additional suggestions:

- Use a heavier grade of rope than ordinary clothesline. This will help you develop a more confident sense of rhythm and coordination. If you stand on the center of the rope, ideally the handles should come up to around your armpits.
- Find a floor that's made out of wood. Don't jump on concrete or even carpet.
- Overcome the temptation to look at your feet. Stand up straight and react only to the sound of the rope hitting the ground.
- Be light and fantastic. Don't come down like a clod on your heels. Practice coming down only on the balls of your feet.

O) Tennis, Racquetball, Squash (and Softball, Basketball, etc.)

Pros: I'm lumping these together because they're obviously sports, but also because you need at least one other person to get a workout. The big plus is that these are fun and competitive. While you might find an excuse not to exercise when left to your own devices, it's harder to weasel out if you've made a commitment to a partner or a whole team.

Cons: Even professional athletes don't rely on their sports to keep them in top condition. Football, baseball, even tennis players rely on hours of jogging and weight training. While shooting baskets or charging a few line drives will definitely burn off some calories, it won't provide a decent aerobic workout. Even tennis and racquetball, unless you play at a fairly high level, are inadequate because of all the starting and stopping.

Should You Injure a Leg Muscle

To minimize tissue damage and accelerate healing of sprains and muscle pulls, perform the following steps:

1. Stop immediately.
2. Take the weight off the leg.

3. Apply ice wrapped in a towel. (Better yet, always keep a sports compress in the freezer. These are plastic bags filled with a special frozen liquid.)
4. Elevate the leg at least three inches.
5. Keep the ice compress on for ten minutes, then off for ten minutes. Repeat at least two more times.
6. Take aspirin or ibuprofen to counter pain and swelling.
7. Don't apply any brace or compression bandage without the approval of your doctor. By immobilizing the injured area, you can sometimes hinder the body's recuperative powers.
8. Simple sprains and muscle pulls usually start to improve within forty-eight to seventy-two hours. But should there be increased swelling or pain or any type of deformity present, then contact your doctor as soon as possible.
9. Wait five days and then start doing some gentle stretching exercises with the injured leg. If there's any serious pain, stop. But if the muscle area is just stiff, continue the stretches and slowly increase the range of motion day by day.
10. Make sure your leg is fully recovered before beginning to work out again. On the first day cut the intensity of each exercise by 50 percent. Then raise it by 10 percent each successive day until you return to your previous level of fitness.

CHAPTER 11

Starting Completely at the Bottom

During the post-pregnancy training the lower body definitely needs more work because it houses the larger muscle groups. For this reason legs are a critical area and building a solid foundation there is exceptionally important.

Bodybuilders frequently use the word *superset* to describe multiple sets of repeating exercises. But in the post-pregnancy training program we very rarely engage in this, unless you're performing at a very advanced level. Instead of supersets we will be doing one set of each exercise and then moving right on to the next exercise. The net result is that you have a continuous flow without having the monotony of doing one set and recovering, and then performing the second set.

> Unlike other programs, my basic approach doesn't require repetitive sets. Rather, you'll receive a series of challenging exercises for different muscle groups. This breaks up the boredom and offers an easy transition for each part of the body that's being trained.

Taking the Bite Out of Cellulite

The name *cellulite* was probably coined by the media, but in reality it's just plain old fat. What we're going to do to control these pockets of fat that usually appear on the thighs and buttocks is simply strengthen muscle fibers, which in turn will smooth out the lumpy appearance of the cellulite. Soon after beginning the post-pregnancy training program, your percentage of body fat will shrink and during the process muscle fibers will elongate and multiply, causing the cellulite to shrivel from sight.

Now granted, genetics will still have some effect on the rate of improvement. But my training is vastly superior to creams, gels, and wraps. These are nothing more than quick fixes which just don't last. And on occasion they can make the situation worse by clogging pores or restraining circulation.

Quite often I acquire clients, especially women, after they have gone on strict diets and lost a lot of weight. True, they now have thin legs, but often the skin over the thighs is loose and sometimes even protrudes over the knees. That's why building leg muscularity is absolutely crucial. It's the only sensible method to fully streamline the lower body, ensuring that the flesh on the legs remains taught and lean, not flabby and folded.

LOWER BODY EXERCISES

1. TARGET MUSCLES: QUADRICEPS AND HAMSTRINGS

PRIMARY BENEFITS: Tightens and tones the appearance of the thighs. Gives greater definition to the buttocks.

A) The Marseille Plié

Note: You can use a chair for balance.

1. Stand straight with your feet a little wider than shoulder length. They should be pointed 45 degrees away from each other. Heels are in; toes are pointed out.

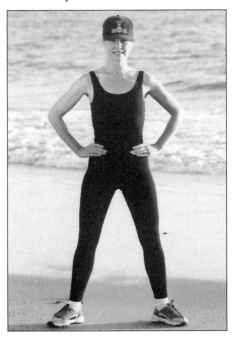

2. Keeping your hands on your waist or holding the back of a chair, start to squat down slowly. Hold the stomach in with your pelvis tucked. Heels and toes should remain on the floor.

3. Come about halfway down. Squeeze your buttocks and inner thigh muscles as you lower yourself. Don't slouch. Make sure to keep your back erect. Your knees should be directly over your toes at a 45-degree angle. *Never* go below a 90-degree bend at the knees.

4. Rise slowly to your starting position and repeat.

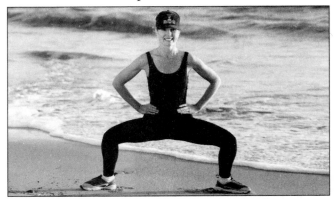

B) Frog Squat

1. Stand with feet slightly apart, heels in, and toes pointed out at a 45-degree angle. Bend down with your fingers on the floor. Keep your feet flat on the floor.

2. Lower yourself until the back of your thighs are almost parallel to the floor. Squeeze the buttocks and inner thighs tightly. Keep the abdomen taut. Your knees should remain above your toes.

3. Straighten your legs until you come back to position #2 and then repeat.

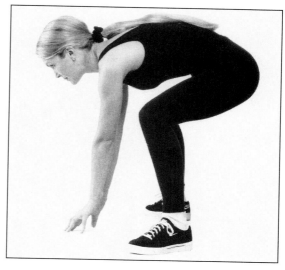

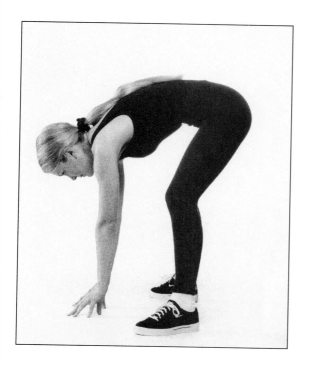

Make sure to always keep your breathing regular. This will help you concentrate and conserve energy.

C) Bent Over Tight Squat

1. Stand with your legs together. The feet should be parallel and pointed forward. Knees are slightly bent as you touch the floor with your fingertips.

2. As if you're sitting, squat down approximately 6 to 12 inches. Squeeze the inner and outer thighs. Keep the feet straight and flat on the floor.

3. Straighten your legs and come back to position #2 and repeat.

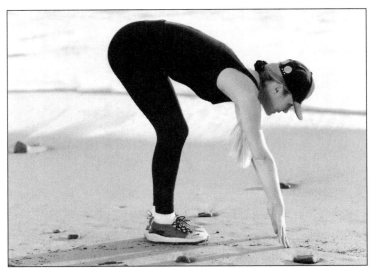

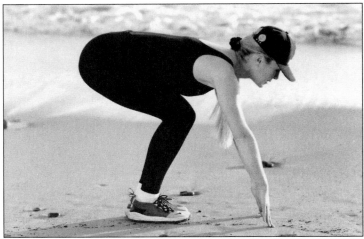

D) Bent Over Marseille Plié

1. Stand with your feet 4 to 6 inches apart. Heels are in; toes are pointed out at 45-degree angles. Knees are slightly bent, in line with your toes. Lower yourself until the back of your thighs are almost parallel to the floor.

2. Bent at the waist and touch your fingers to the floor. This position is very similar to the Frog Squat except here your feet are much closer together. Squeeze your buttocks and inner thighs tightly. Keep the abdomen taut. Make sure your knees stay over your toes.

3. Straighten your legs until you come back to starting position and repeat.

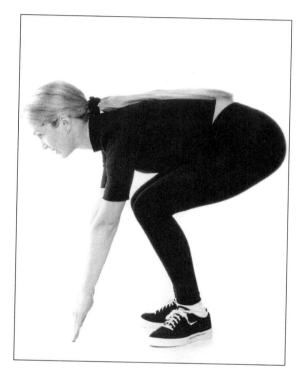

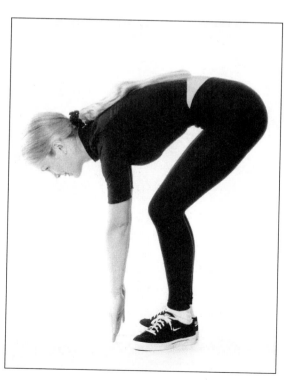

In the beginning, working out three times during the week is a safe and realistic approach. Of course, later on you can do more if you wish. The choice is always yours.

E) Standing Squat

1. Stand with legs together; feet are straight and parallel to each other.
2. Bend the knees 90 degrees until the back of your thighs are parallel to the floor. Now pretend you're sitting in a chair. But as you descend let your arms extend straight forward to shoulder height. Heels should stay on the floor. Body and shoulders are erect.

3. Rise slowly from your sitting position. As you do, squeeze the back of your legs and your buttocks. Don't let your knees flay out. Avoid slumping forward.

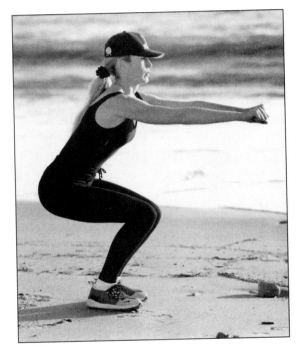

F) Skiing Squat

1. Crouch down slightly as if you were skiing with knees bent and feet pointed forward, four to six inches apart. Your arms are in praying position.
2. Bend down at the knee six inches. Keep your feet on the floor and parallel to each other. Keep your upper thighs and lower calf muscles contracted.
3. Rise to starting position and repeat.

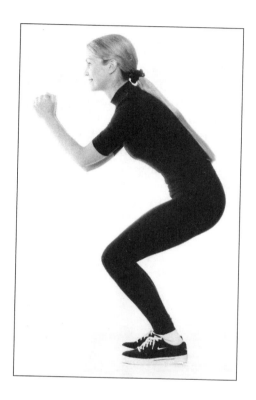

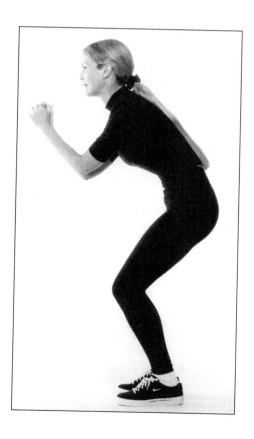

Although it's tempting, don't start off with a bang. Work easily at your own pace. By slowly increasing the intensity over weeks and months, you won't become frustrated.

G) Step-ups: Alternating

1. Stand before a bench or stair six to eight inches high. Feet are parallel and pointed forward.
2. Step up with the right foot followed by the left. Make sure your foot lands squarely on the step. Your body should be erect. If you choose you may pump your arms while performing this.
3. Step down with the right foot followed by the left.
4. Step up with your left foot followed by your right.
5. Step down with your left foot followed by your right.
6. Start again with your right foot and repeat.

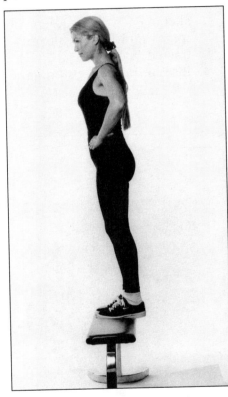

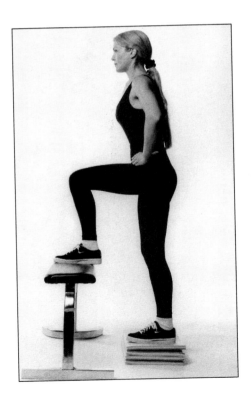

Avoid erratic exercise schedules. Don't exercise twice one week and make up for it by working out four times the next week. This confuses the body and can result in stress injuries.

H) Step-ups: Single Leg (Right)

1. Stand before an elevated surface six to eight inches high. Feet are parallel and pointed forward.
2. Put your right foot on top of it, keeping the left foot on the floor.
3. Bring up your left foot and touch the back of the bench or stair with your left toe. Most of the lifting should be performed by the right leg. Keep your back erect.
4. Lower the left foot to the floor and repeat.

Single Leg (Left)

1. Now put the right foot on the floor and the left one on top of the elevated surface.
2. Bring up your right foot and touch the back of the bench or stair with your right toe. Most of the lifting should be performed by the left leg. Again, keep your back erect.
3. Lower the left leg to the floor and repeat.

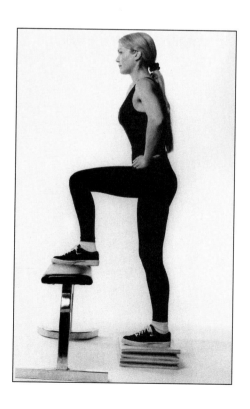

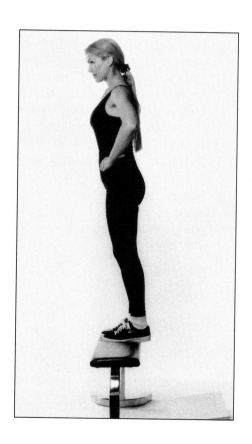

I) Alternate Lunges

1. Stand with your feet four to six inches apart and hands on your hips. Keeping the toes pointed straight ahead, step back with the left foot. The distance from the back of your right heel to your left toes should be two and a half feet.
2. Keeping your left foot straight, slowly bend the right knee as far as you can go, coming up on the left toe. Depending on your flexibility, the angle of your right leg should be between 45 and 90 degrees. Make sure your back is straight.
3. Slowly straighten your right leg. Bring your left leg forward so that it is now parallel with your right. Place your right leg back two and a half to three feet. Bend your left leg and now perform the exercise on that side.
4. Slowly straighten the left leg. Bring your right leg forward to the starting position. Repeat.

J) Single Leg Lunges

1. Take the same starting position as the alternate lunge.
2. Perform on the right side without alternating legs.
3. Perform equal number on the left side without alternating legs.

Never stop abruptly! This can cause dizziness, faintness, or nausea from inadequate blood supply. If you're getting overly fatigued, slowly wind down the exercise routine and perform a few light stretches.

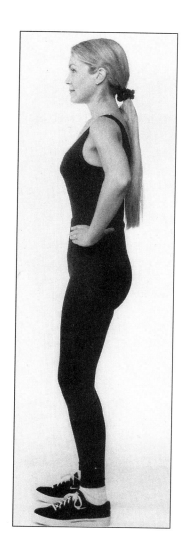

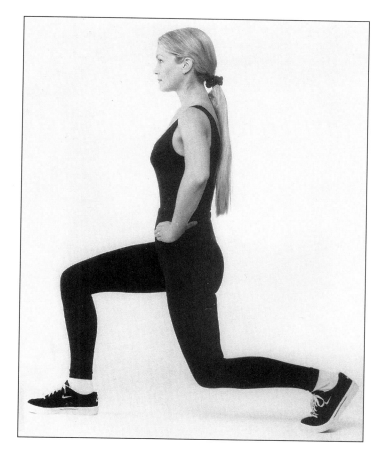

K) Bench Lunges

1. Stand about 2 1/2 feet away from a bench or a block that is about 4 to 6 inches high; your back is to the bench. Put your hands on your hips.
2. Place your right instep flat on the elevated surface; your lower leg is parallel to the floor.
3. Slowly bend your left leg; your right knee bends toward the floor.

4. Return to position #2 and repeat. When you lunge your repetitions perform an equal number of reps with your left foot on the bench.

If you're too exhausted for a strenuous workout, don't worry about it. Just do some easy stretches instead. You'll keep your resolve as well as keep your muscles warm and limber.

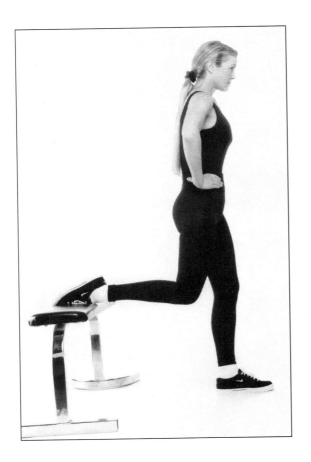

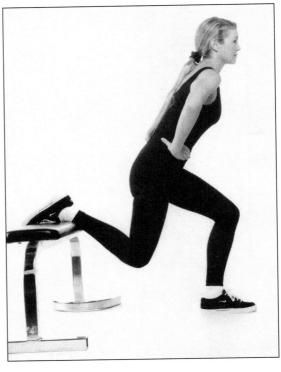

2. TARGET MUSCLES: GLUTES, ADDUCTORS, AND ABDUCTORS

PRIMARY BENEFITS: Uplift the buttocks and eliminate flab. Strengthen, slim, and shape the thighs, both front and back.

L) Flutter Kicks

1. Lie down on your stomach. Legs are straight and toes extended. As if you were swimming, raise your right leg from the hip. Squeeze the right buttock. Don't bend the knee.
2. Allow the motion to elevate the hip about 2 to 4 inches above the floor.
3. Bring the right leg down. As you do, raise the left leg, lifting from the hip.
4. Lower it and repeat.

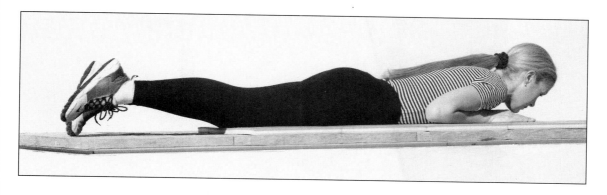

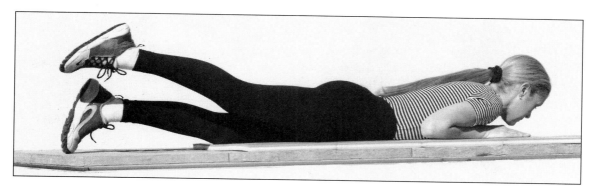

M) Glute Raises

1. Get down on all fours.
2. Raise your right leg so that your thigh is parallel with the floor and your knee is bent 90 degrees. Make sure your toes are pointed straight behind you.
3. Raise your leg 2 to 4 inches above the parallel position. Keep the knee bent.
4. Lower leg to the position in step #2.
5. After completion, do the same number of reps on left side.

Let me again emphasize that replacing fluids is absolutely vital. Have a good supply of water close at hand. For every half hour of intense activity, you will need a full glass of water. Naturally, the warmer the weather, the more you should drink.

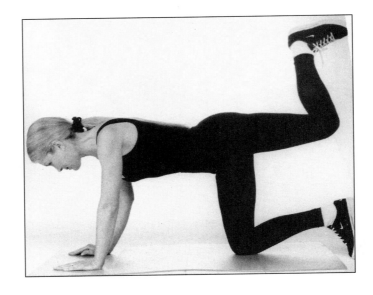

N) Pelvic Thrusts

1. Lie flat on your back with your knees bent and legs and feet together. Keep your feet pointed straight ahead. Put a hand beneath each buttock.
2. Now lift your pelvis as high as it can go, simultaneously squeezing your buttocks.

3. Return to starting position.

Set up a regular exercise schedule. Always be prepared to allot a specific time for working out, whether it's first thing in the morning, over lunch, late in the afternoon, or even after dinner.

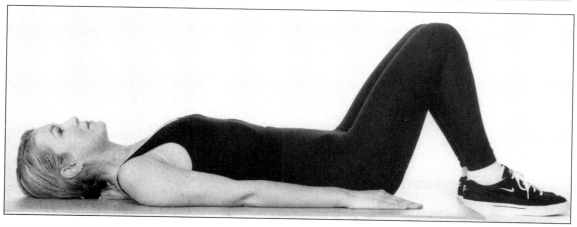

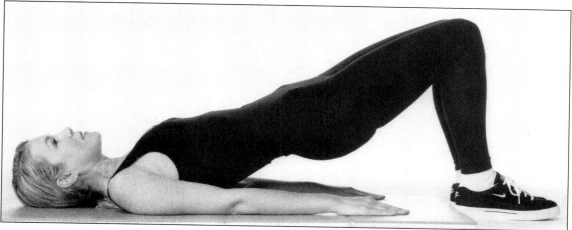

O) Lateral Leg Lifts (Straight)

1. Lie on the floor on your right side. Your left hip should be slightly rotated forward. The right leg is bent at a 90-degree angle to the stomach and the left leg is straight, the foot touching the floor.
2. Raise the right leg from the floor to right hip level. Do not lift higher than the hip.
3. Return right leg to starting position. Repeat.
4. Do same number of reps lying on your left side.

During winter you may be tempted to slack off. But maintaining your fitness level is critical, especially at this time of the year. Continuing to exercise strengthens your immune system, allowing you to more powerfully ward off colds and the flu.

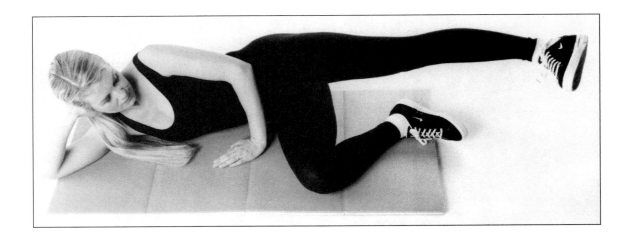

P) Lateral Leg Lifts (45 Degrees)

1. Lie on the floor on your right side. The left leg is held at a 45-degree angle and the left foot is elevated about 6 inches above the floor. The right leg is bent 90 degrees.

2. Lift the left leg another 6 inches.
3. Bring it back down to position #1. Repeat.
4. Do same number of reps lying on your left side.

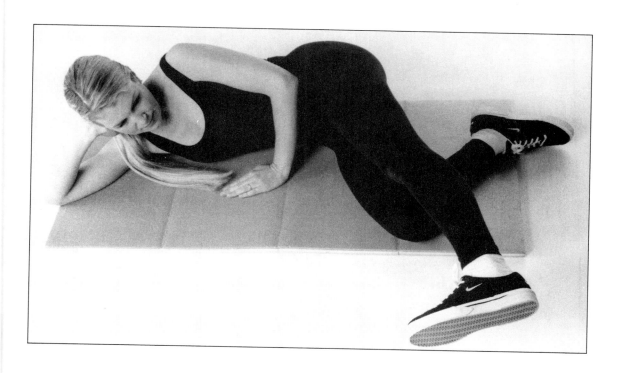

Q) Lateral Leg Lifts (90 Degrees)

1. Lie on the floor on your right side. The left leg is held at a 90-degree angle to the body and the left foot is elevated about 6 inches. The right leg is bent 90 degrees.

2. Lift the left leg another 6 inches.
3. Bring it back down to position #1. Repeat.
4. Do same number of reps lying on your left side.

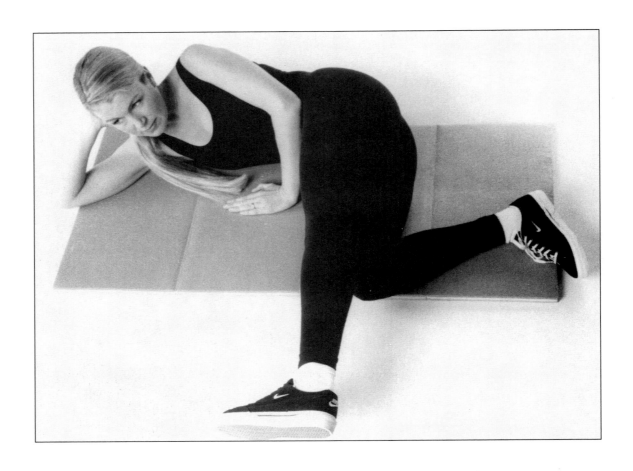

R) Kick Outs

1. Lie on the floor on your right side. Both knees are bent 90 degrees. Elevate the left leg 45 degrees from your hip.
2. Pushing out with the heel, kick out straight with the left leg. Foot is flexed.
3. Bring leg back to position #1. Repeat.

4. Do same number of reps lying on your right side.

Should you discover that your mind is drifting while exercising, gently coach it back. Stop a moment and refocus on exactly what you're doing and why. By staying in the present, you're giving yourself the present of maximum fitness.

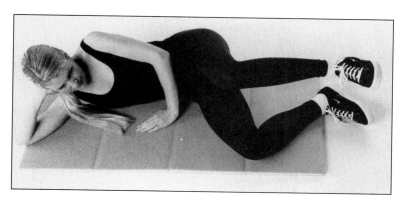

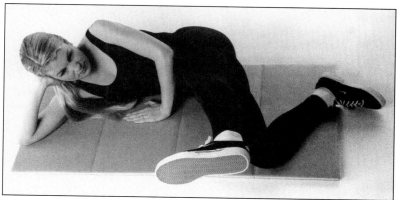

S) Inner Thigh Lift

1. Lie on your right side. Bend the left leg at the knee and bring the left foot over the right leg to rest on the floor. The right leg should remain straight with the foot flexed.
2. Slowly raise the right leg 6 inches or to the highest possible point.

3. Return to starting position.
4. After completion, repeat same number of reps lying on the left side to work the left leg.

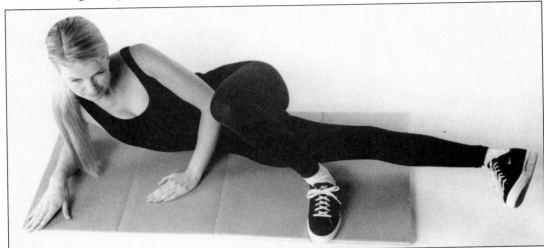

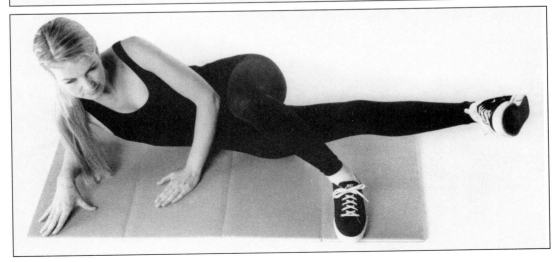

T) Inner Thigh Lift with Bench

1. Lie on your right side. The left leg should be straight and resting on top of an elevated surface such as a bench, no less than 8 inches above the floor and no higher than comfortable. The right leg should be straight as well.

2. Keeping it straight, raise the right leg to touch the bench or elevated surface.
3. Return to starting position.
4. After completion, do the same number of reps on the left side working the left leg.

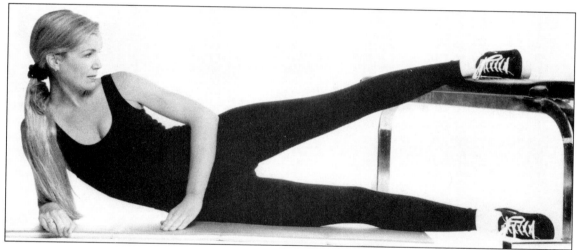

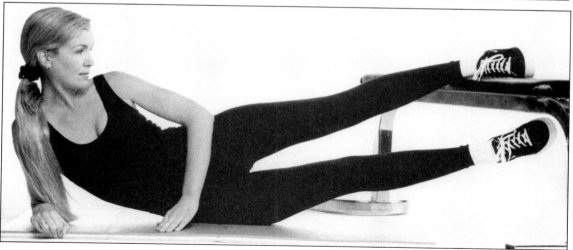

3. ISOLATION EXERCISES FOR THE LEGS

PRIMARY BENEFITS: Defines and tones the muscles of the calves and thighs individually.

U) Leg Extension

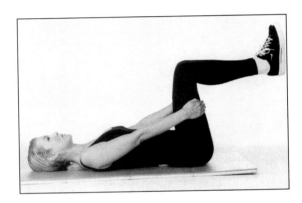

1. Lie on your back with legs together. Lift your legs with knees bent 90 degree and calves parallel to the floor. Hold the back of your thighs for support.
2. Extend your legs straight in the air, making sure not to lock knees. Squeeze your front thigh muscles as tightly as possible.
3. Return to starting position and repeat.

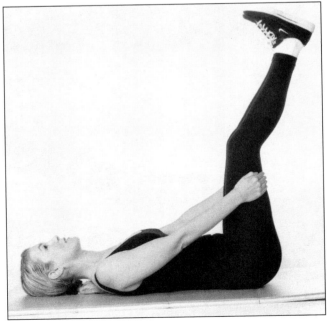

V) Leg Curls

1. Lie flat on the floor or upon a mat facedown. Legs should be straight and together. Rest your head on your hands.
2. Bend your right leg 90 degrees at the knee. Squeeze your back and thigh muscles as tightly as possible as you raise your foot.

3. Return to starting position and repeat.
4. Perform the same number of reps with the left leg.

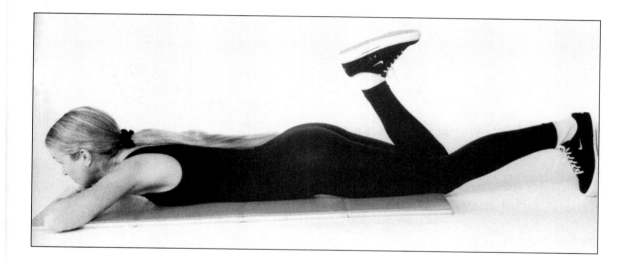

Instantly stop exercising if you develop pain anywhere, particularly in your knees, hips, pelvis, shoulders, or ankles. If the pain persists after stopping—or recurs during your next workout—see a physician. My advice is never try to diagnose yourself.

W) Basic Calf Raise

1. Stand erect on a block or step. You can lean your hands against a wall or hold a rail for support. The weight should be on the balls of your feet, and your heels should be over the edge. Your feet should be parallel and together.
2. Raise up on the balls of your feet as far as you can go. Hold for one second and slowly lower yourself. Your heels should go below the level of the top of the block.
3. Return to starting position and repeat.

X) Calf Raise—Heels In/Toes Out

1. Stand on a block or step as in Basic Calf Raise. But this time your heels are placed inward at 45 degrees to each other with your toes pointed out.
2. Raise up on the balls of your feet as far as you can go. Hold for one second and slowly lower yourself. Your heels should go below the level of the top of the block.
3. Return to starting position and repeat.

Y) Calf Raise—Toes In/Heels Out

1. Stand on a block or step as in the Basic Calf Raise. But this time your toes are placed inward at 45 degrees to each other with your heels pointed out.
2. Raise up on the balls of your feet as far as you can go. Hold for one second and slowly lower yourself. Your heels should go below the level of the top of the block.
3. Return to starting position and repeat.

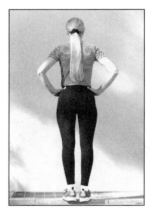

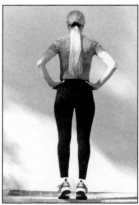

CHAPTER 12

Getting into Top Shape

Many men are preoccupied with their upper bodies and just as many women are not, which is extremely unfortunate in both cases. Women generally tend to concentrate or their lower halves, their thighs and abdominal areas in particular. Nevertheless it's imperative that a balanced approach be taken for both the upper and lower body, because if one section is underdeveloped, it will definitely detract from the other. Working the upper body during the post-pregnancy training not only produces striking definition, but creates a sense of bearing which is both youthful and confidant. Most of these exercises will require the use of weights.

PLEASE NOTE: The amount of weight you will be using will vary with the level of training you're working at. For my specific recommendations, consult Chapter Eight.

UPPER-BODY EXERCISES

1. TARGET MUSCLES: BICEPS, DELTOIDS, TRAPEZIUS, AND LATISSIMUS DORSI

PRIMARY BENEFITS: Strengthening and shaping the back muscles; developing the shoulders; firming and defining the forearms.

Important: Keep your abs tight and your pelvis tucked in for all the following exercises. Keep both shoulders back and level. Chest should be out. Don't allow your body to droop forward or backward.

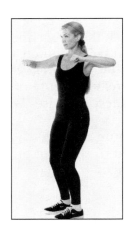 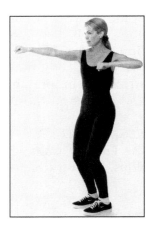

> After each weight-lifting exercise, give yourself adequate time to recover. Don't rush into the next phase without first resting for a few moments to catch your breath.

A) Power Punch

1. Stand up straight with feet shoulder width apart. Arms are extended forward and away from the body at shoulder height and flexed 90 degrees at the elbows. Fists are clenched. Forearms are parallel with the floor.
2. Punch the right arm fully toward a spot directly in front of you. Pull back the arm and follow with a punch with the left arm to the same spot.
3. Put a lot of snap and focus into each punch you throw.

> Never compare your performance to that of others, especially those considerably more adept at training and working out. This only serves to make you more critical of yourself. What's more, it tends to make you overlook all the great progress you've already made.

B) Alternate Military Press

1. Stand up straight with feet shoulder width apart. Arms are perpendicular to the body and bent at the elbows 90 degrees. Palms are facing out. Elbows are parallel to the floor.
2. Punch upward with the right hand. Pull the arm back and then punch upward with the left.
3. Make the movement powerful and the extension full.

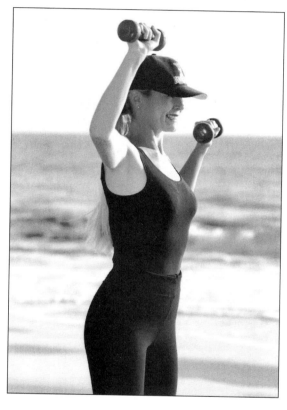

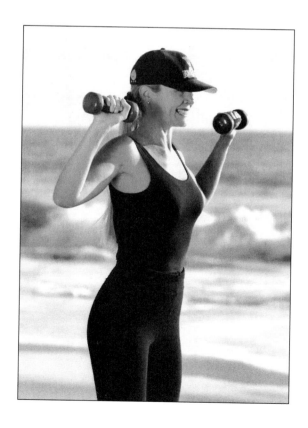

C) Backstrokes

1. Stand up straight with feet shoulder width apart. Arms are straight at your sides.
2. Raise the right arm up and back and then follow with the left, using an alternating movement as if you were swimming. Be certain that the only rotation occurs at the shoulders.
3. Make the motion full and sweeping.

D) Arm Circles

1. Stand up straight with feet shoulder width apart. Hold your arms straight out to the sides. Palms should be facing down toward the floor.
2. Create tight 6-inch circles as you rotate your arms forward from the shoulders.
3. Complete the reps and then face your palms upward.
4. Now create tight 6-inch circles as you rotate your arms backward from the shoulders, doing the same number of reps as you did forward.

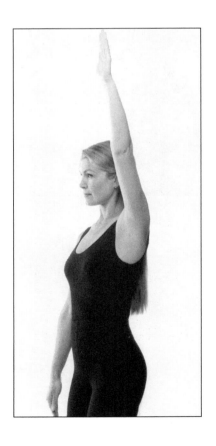

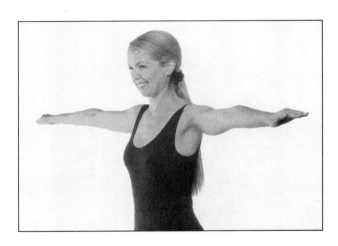

If you can't do twenty repetitions, do fifteen; if not fifteen, then ten. No amount is too small. In fact, just doing one is a thousand percent better than doing none; because doing nothing takes you nowhere.

E) Shoulder Shrugs

1. Stand up straight with feet shoulder width apart. Arms are straight at your sides, palms facing hips. Now sag your shoulders forward and downward as far as possible.

2. Slowly shrug your shoulder upward as high as possible and backward as far as possible.
3. Return to starting position and repeat.

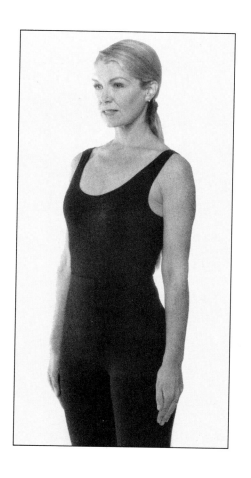

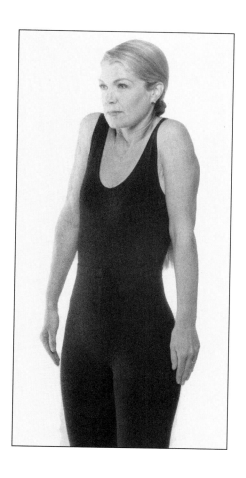

F) Seated Lat Rows

1. Sit on a bench or chair. Feet are together.
2. Bring chest down to your thighs. Palms should be facing each other and are down around the ankles. Elbows are close to knees.

3. Raise your elbows as far back as you can, pinching your shoulder blades. Both elbows and arms should be kept as close to your rib cage as possible.
4. Slowly lower arms to position #2 and complete reps.

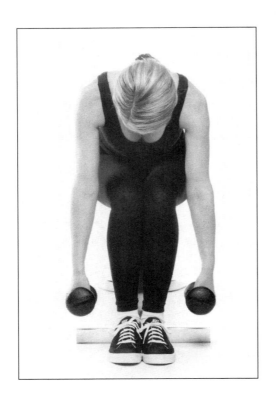 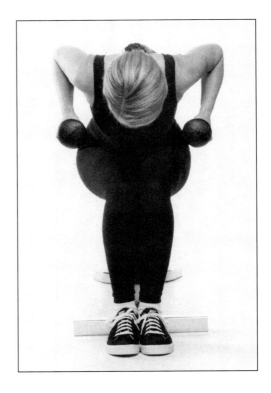

G) Seated Rows

1. Sit on a bench or chair. Feet are together.
2. Bring chest down to your thighs. Palms are facing back and are down by your ankles. Elbows are close to the knees.
3. Using a rowing motion, bring elbows upward until the shoulder blades pinch.
4. Slowly lower and complete reps.

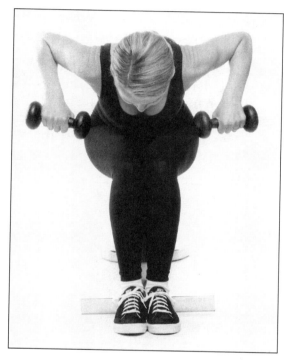

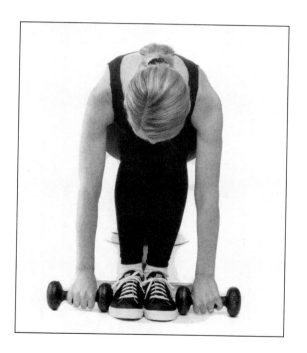

Once again, let me emphasize that you have to work both the right and left sides evenly. The same amount of repetitions must be done with both arms—as well as both legs. By balancing your strength exercises, you create a beautiful sense of physical symmetry and poise.

H) Hammer Curl

1. You can perform this exercise either standing or seated. Feet are shoulder width apart and parallel. Arms are running straight down your sides. Palms are always facing inward.

2. Slowly curl the weights up to your shoulders. (This may be done with both hands at once or one hand at a time.) The upper arm shoulder remains still as you flex only at the elbows.

3. Lower the weights to the starting position and complete reps. (If you are using one hand at a time, an equal number of reps must be performed on both sides.)

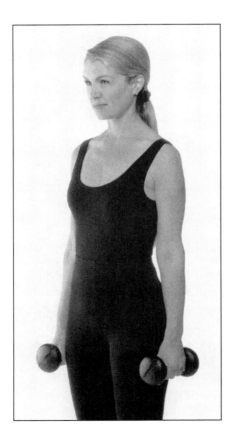

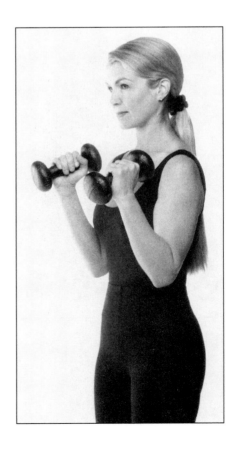

I) Hammer Curl with Twist

1. Stand with feet parallel and slightly more than shoulder length apart. Keep your back straight. Your palms are facing your legs.
2. Keeping your upper arms motionless, slowly curl the weights upward. About halfway up rotate the palms so that they are now facing the ceiling.
3. On the way down slowly reverse the movement so that the palms wind up facing the legs again. Repeat.

Avoid placing unnecessary mental burdens on yourself. Never say that you "need to" work out. Nor think that you "have to" or "ought to" exercise. Instead substitute positive phrases such as "I want to" get in shape; "I prefer" being slim and taut; "I wish" to be healthier, etc.

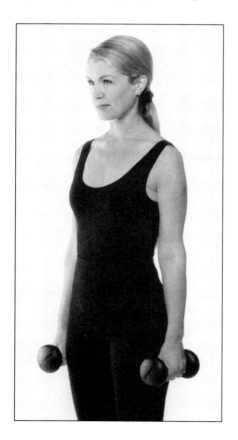

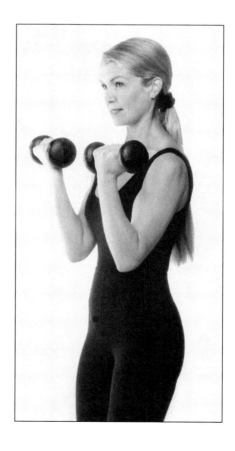

J) Sprint Curls

1. Stand with feet parallel and shoulder width apart. Your torso is shifted slightly forward, bent at the waist. Palms are facing each other and elbows are locked at 90 degrees, close to the rib cage.
2. Raise the right weight and then lower it.
3. Raise the left weight and then lower it.

4. Keep alternating back and forth. Make the movements intense and powerful, twisting the torso as if you were running fast. Repeat.

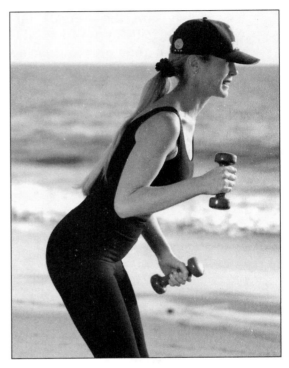

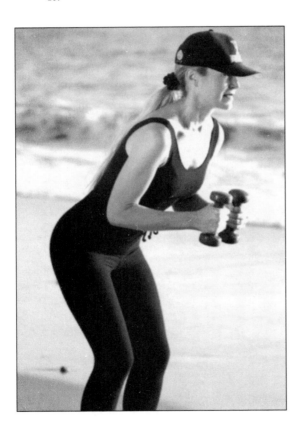

It's important to remember that what you want to achieve is a process of small steps. Don't give yourself rigid time limits for losing weight or reaching a certain level of fitness. Working out is always a win-win situation. As long as you continue, you can't lose.

2. TARGET MUSCLES: PECTORALS, DELTOIDS, AND TRICEPS

PRIMARY BENEFITS: Developing and strengthening the chest; defining and shaping the forearms.

Important: An exercise should be done one movement after the other with no rest in between.

K) Push-ups

Note: Depending upon your level of strength and fitness, choose *one* of the following three positions. Push-ups on the knees are the easiest, with each position getting progressively more difficult. Always keep your head even with your chest; don't let it droop down. Always make sure your abs are tight and your back straight.

1. On Knees

1. Get down on all fours. Knees are bent and hands are shoulder width apart on the floor. Buttocks are up. Legs are parallel on the floor.
2. Bend the elbows. Chest drops and touches the floor. Shoulders are over hands.
3. Push up by extending arms. Keep back straight. Repeat.

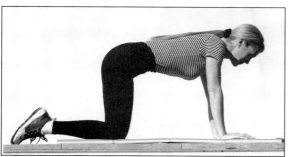

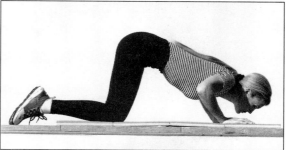

2. Incline

1. Lean against a sturdy table, chair, or wall at a 45-degree angle. Keep your body straight and stand on your toes.
2. Bend the elbows and drop your chest toward the table or chair or wall.
3. Push up by extending arms. Repeat.

Don't expect to get back to your "old self" overnight. It will take at least several months, so don't rush yourself.

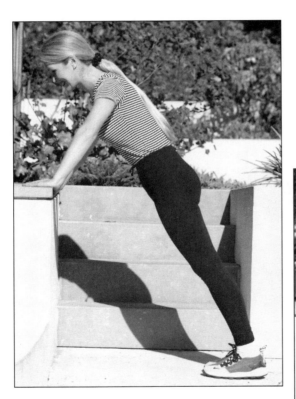

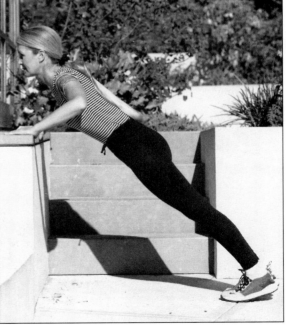

3. *Standard*

1. Rest on your hands and toes. Hands are shoulder width apart, legs are held parallel.
2. Bend elbows and drop chest to floor. Arms should be bent at 90 degrees. Don't let the back arch downward.
3. Push up by extending the arms. Repeat.

It doesn't pay to wait for encouragement from others. The first thing is to always give it to yourself. For example, buy yourself a little present or keepsake for meeting a specific goal or fitness level—even if it's only doing five more sit-ups. Be proud of what you've achieved. Bask in the glow. After all, the loudest applause comes from inside.

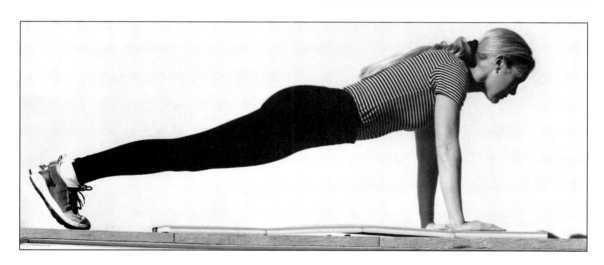

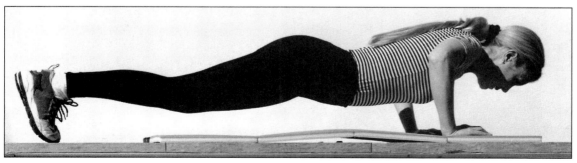

L) Anterior Windmills

1. Stand with feet shoulder width apart. Arms are at your sides with palms facing back. Abs are tight. Pelvis is tucked.

2. Starting with your right arm, alternately bring your arms back and around, using the largest circular motion you possibly can. Imagine that you're swimming, doing the crawlstroke.

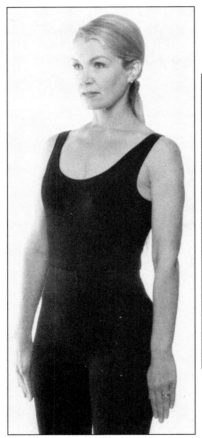

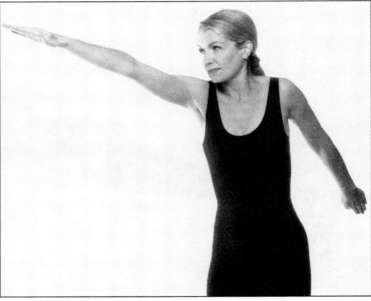

M) Pec Push

1. Stand with feet shoulder width apart. Elbows are held up to shoulder level and bent at 90 degrees. Upper arms should be parallel to floor; palms are facing forward.

2. Squeeze the arms together making a *U* with the forearms.
3. Slowly bring back to starting position. Repeat.

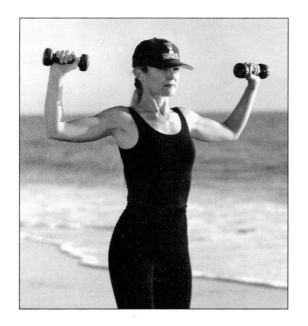

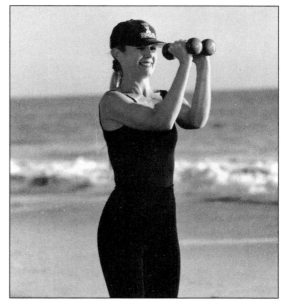

N) Tight Pec Squeeze

1. Stand with feet shoulder width apart. Arms are extended straight out in front, shoulder width apart.
2. Cross the right wrist *over* the left wrist keeping arms straight and un-cross back to starting position.
3. Cross the right wrist *under* the left wrist and uncross back to starting position.
4. Keep repeating steps 2 and 3.

Sometimes there are negative thoughts floating around in your mind. Many of these come from way back in childhood. However, if you sustain this exercise program, the incredible self-esteem that results often allows you to laugh these very same thoughts right out of your head.

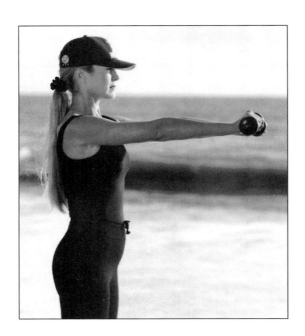

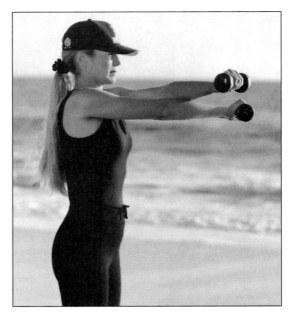

O) Prone Bench Press

Note: If you don't have a bench or an equivalent surface, lie on the floor, although this will impede your motions somewhat.

1. Lie flat on the bench. Knees are bent with your feet resting on the edge of the bench. If it is more comfortable, you can keep your feet on the floor. Dumbbells are held chest high with elbows bent at a 90-degree angle. Palms are facing front. (If you are on the floor, elbows are out to the sides with hands positioned over elbows.)

2. Extend the arms upward, keeping your back straight and flat on the bench.
3. Slowly lower dumbbells to starting position. Repeat.

Note: To intensify this exercise, *substitute* the following:

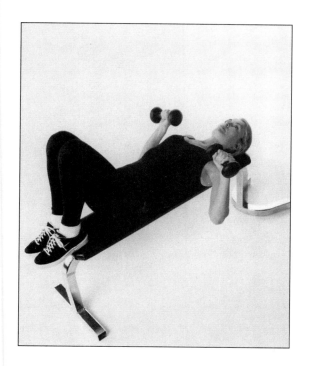

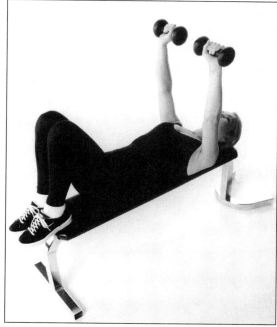

With Twist

1. Same starting position as above.
2. Fully extend the arms upward. As you do, twist your arms so that your palms face each other and the dumbbells touch.
3. Slowly lower the dumbbells to the starting position. While performing this, twist your arms back so that the palms are facing each other once more. Repeat.

Your breathing should always be deep and regular, never those shallow little inhales that can rob your body of oxygen and make you lightheaded or dizzy. Feel your chest expand and shoulders rise with every breath.

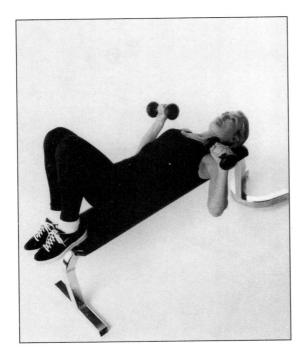

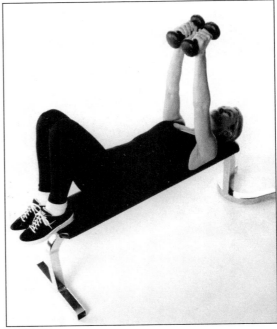

P) Super Flyes

1. Lie prone on a flat exercise bench. Feet are flat on the bench or the floor for support.
2. Extend the arms straight upward and lift the dumbbells over your head so that they are directly above your shoulder joints. Make sure your wrists are facing each other. Bend your elbows slightly.
3. Slowly lower the dumbbells in a semicircular arc as far down as you can. Elbows should wind up below the level of your torso. Be certain to keep your elbows bent at all times.

4. Extend the arms upward until the dumbbells have reached the position in step #2. Repeat.

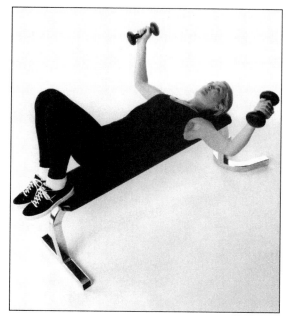

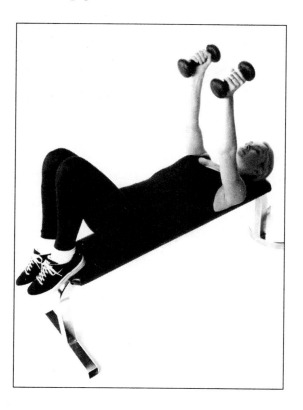

By sticking to a workout schedule you'll notice other powerful changes in your life. Stress will be lessened and you'll be solving problems more thoroughly. But remember, it all starts with that special commitment to yourself. So no excuses for not training!

Q) Reverse Super Flyes

1. Lie prone on a flat exercise bench. Feet are flat on the bench or the floor for support.
2. Hold dumbbells straight outward with elbows slightly bent. (Weights should be lighter or eliminated for this exercise.)
3. Bring the dumbbells together directly over the center of your chest. Keep your back straight and flat on the bench.
4. Slowly lower the dumbbells to the #2 position. Repeat.

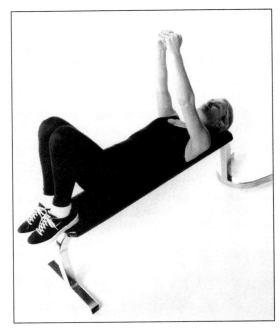

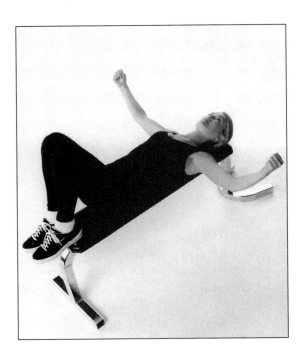

R) Tricep Kickbacks

1. Stand with your legs 46 inches apart, knees bent and your torso shifted slightly forward.
2. Arms are bent 45 degrees with palms facing each other. Keep arms tight to the body. For the rest of the exercise the upper arms *never* move.
3. Extend your arms back as far as they can go. Hold a moment.
4. Slowly bring the arm back to the position in step #2. Repeat.

If your weight hasn't changed much, don't worry. It probably has to do with biological factors such as fluctuations in water retention, which frequently shifts due to sodium consumption and menstrual cycles. More to the point, ask yourself how you're feeling on a day-to-day basis. That's the real test of success.

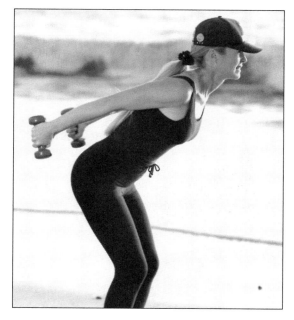

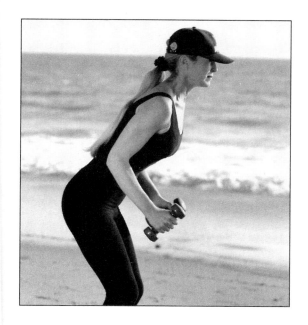

S) Tricep Dips

1. Grip the front edge of a bench or step with your palms facing backward. Hands should be a little wider than shoulder length apart. Knees are bent 90 degrees, feet and legs are together. Back is straight.
2. Bend your arms as much as possible, lowering your buttocks to the floor. Keep your back close to the bench. (To increase the intensity, you may place a light dumbbell in your lap.)
3. Push slowly back upward to the starting position. Repeat.

Always perform the exercises slowly and deliberately. Trying to race through the routines not only taxes your cardiovascular system, but increases the risk of injury due to improper form.

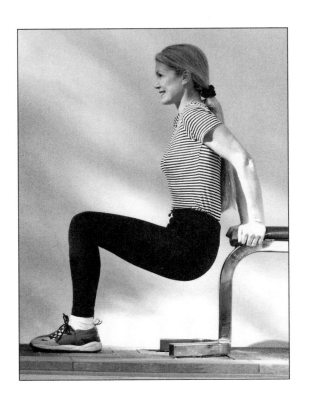
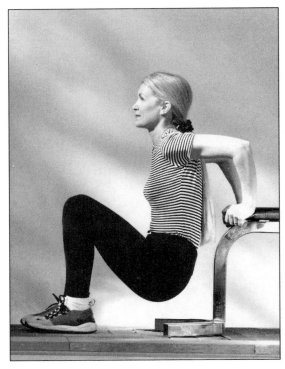

T) Curls to Military Press

1. Stand with feet shoulder width apart. The pelvis is tucked and the abs are tight; arms straight at your sides, palms facing your body.
2. Bend your elbows, curling the dumbbells upward until they reach shoulder level.
3. Now straighten your arms, raising the dumbbells above your head. Don't allow your torso to bend backward. Keep the back straight.
4. Slowly lower the dumbbells back down to shoulder level.
5. Pause for a moment. And then slowly lower the dumbbells down to starting position and repeat.

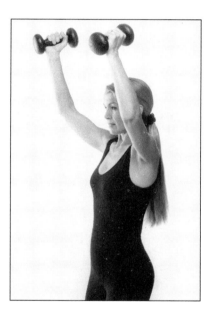

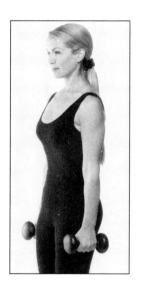

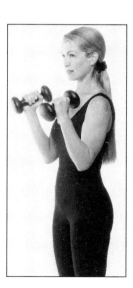

Naturally any illness or emergency can interrupt your exercise schedule for a couple of weeks or more. Should this happen, picking up where you left off might cause injury, so lessen the weight you've been using. Always allow your body enough time to recover before returning to your previous level.

U) Bicep Curls

1. Stand up straight with feet shoulder width apart. Arms are straight at your sides, held close against the torso. Palms are facing your body.
2. Bend your elbows, curling the dumbbells up to your shoulder.
3. Lower arms to starting position and repeat.

Check your pulse rate five minutes after completing each phase of your workout. If it is over 100 beats a minute, you've been pushing yourself too hard. Cut back on the intensity of your exercise program. You've probably been attempting too much too soon.

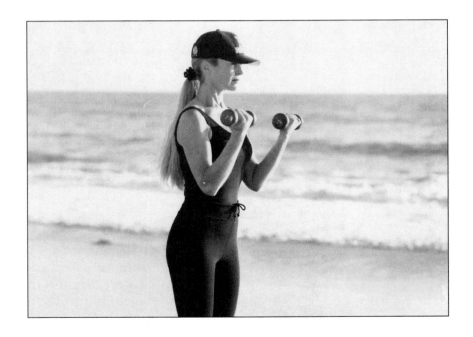

CHAPTER 13

Streamlining the Stomach

The process of giving birth immediately results in the loss of about twelve pounds. Even so, most women find this of small comfort, particularly if they've gained twenty-five pounds or more. Upon gazing at their postpartum reflections in the mirror, they can witness protruding abdomens caused by their still enlarged uterus.

But the good news is that the uterus will contract to its pre-pregnancy size within six weeks. Nevertheless, the muscles in the abdomen have probably weakened, stretched out and sagged, meaning a concerted effort must be made in order to get the flat, tight stomach you want.

Therefore, in order to tighten up that drooping abdomen, you can start working out as soon as 72 hours after giving birth—provided your delivery was normal and uncomplicated. But if surgery was involved or some other form of delivery trauma, then you must consult with your physician before commencing.

CAUTION: Don't attempt any of the following until you are certain that the recti abdominis (a pair of muscles which line your abdominal area) aren't detached from each other. This separation (also known as diastasis) is not unusual among women who've had several children. Unless this muscular rift is completely healed, it can be aggravated by even moderate exercise. Ask your nurse or physician if you suspect this condition.

Getting a Washboard Stomach

Some women believe that doing a thousand sit-ups a day will result in a washboard stomach. Well, that's simply not the case. Abdominal work requires quality, not quantity, so don't get wrapped up in a large number of reps. What I strive for is ten to fifteen minutes of focused and intensive abdominal work. The proper form is more important than the number of reps you do. To realize an effective and efficient workout, good, precise movements are the key.

Another reason to focus on abdominal work is the prevention of lower back pain. Women in particular are susceptible to this common affliction both during and after pregnancy. Lower back pain can become chronic and cost a small fortune, not only in lost productivity but in doctors' and chiropractors' bills as well. The truth is, the vast majority of lower back pain is easily preventible and in many cases completely reversible; but this doesn't happen by working your back—only by working your front, your stomach muscles.

For most individuals suffering from chronic back pain, physiological research has shown that their abdominal muscles are only about one third as strong as the muscles in their back. Bulging bellies start after having a child when stomach muscles start to soften and sag, weakening the entire area and causing the abdomen to protrude.

Consequently, to compensate for much of this post-pregnant weight hanging over the waistline, the burden of support is shifted to the back. From there your pelvis leans forward and your butt sticks out. As a result of being so bent out of shape, the bottom joints along the spine eventually demand even more muscle tension to support them.

Ultimately, those same muscles weary of all this increased stress and pressure, and suddenly you're lying flat on your back, or simply wishing you were. Without question, the best way to rid yourself of lower back pain is through abdominal conditioning. The following exercises will not only pull in your gut, but your butt as well.

ABDOMINAL EXERCISES

1. TARGET MUSCLES: UPPER AND LOWER ABDOMINALS; EXTERNAL OBLIQUES; INTERCOSTALS

PRIMARY BENEFITS: Tightens and tones the appearance of the stomach. Realigns and lifts the buttocks.

Important: You must wait at least four weeks after giving birth before attempting any full sit-ups, knee-chest routines, or double leg lifts.

> **Always exhale fully when contracting your abdominal muscles and inhale as you expand them.**

A) Sit-ups

1. Start by lying on your back on a mat on the floor or on an abdominal board. Bend your knees slightly and rest your heels on the floor. Extend your arms in front of you, with your fingers pointing straight ahead.

2. Begin lifting your head and upper shoulders using your abdominal muscles, bringing your hands between your knees. Be sure to keep your lower back flat on the floor.

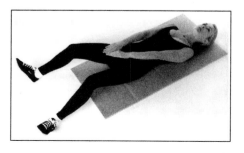

3. Keeping your stomach muscles tight, lower yourself to the starting position.

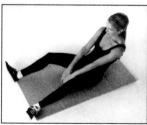

> Working out is your private time and should be completely respected by those around you. You are not being self-centered or selfish by focusing on fitness. Rather, you are ensuring that you will be healthy and stress-free for the sake of your family.

B) Crunchy Crunches

Note: In the beginning you may wish to put a pillow in between your knees, especially if you've had a cesarean.

1. Lying on the floor, bend your legs with your feet flat on the floor. Hands are placed behind your head.
2. Contract your stomach muscles and raise your head and shoulders off the floor. Do not put forward pressure on your head with your hands. As you continue the motion, raise your knees to your elbows. Use your lower abdomen muscles to raise your hips off the floor, but make sure your lower back remains flat and does not arch.

3. When you come up as far as you can, hold the position for two seconds, then slowly lower yourself back down. Repeat.

Note: You may vary this exercise by leaning your legs straight up against a wall perpendicular to the floor.

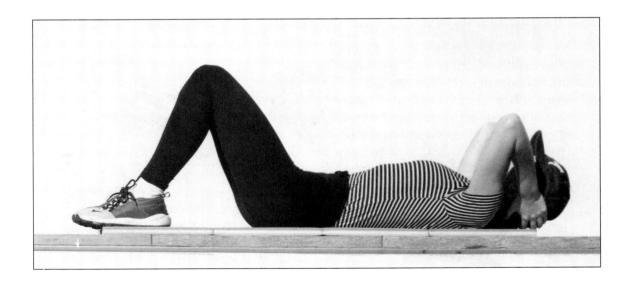

Each one of these abdominal exercises will help diminish the chance of varicose veins, backaches, and leg cramps. They will greatly lessen the odds of you developing edema or blood clots in the veins (technically known as thrombi). And because of the improvement in blood circulation, any trauma to the uterus, abdomen, and pelvic regions will be mended much faster.

If during exercising you experience difficulty in standing, headaches, loss of muscle control, or palpitations, stop right there. Sit down and take a few deep breaths. Talk to your doctor and make certain that you have no underlying conditions that could hamper your progress.

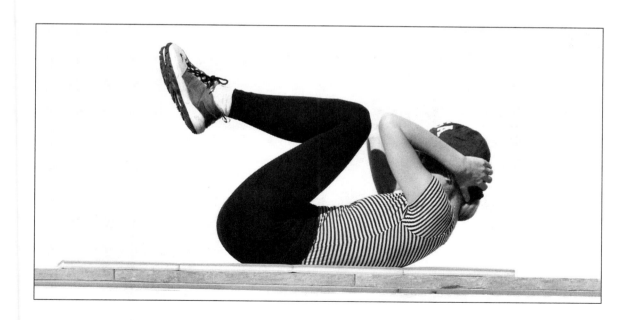

C) Alternate Elbows to Knees

1. Lie on the floor or on a gym bench with your knees bent at a 45-degree angle and feet flat on the floor. Hands are placed behind your head with elbows out.
2. As in doing a sit-up, use your abdominal muscles to roll up. At the same time, touch your right elbow to your left knee by twisting your torso. Don't press against your neck or head with your hands.
3. Return to your starting position. Now roll up once more to touch your left elbow to your right knee.
4. Return to your starting position and repeat from the beginning.

> Always make sure that your abdominal muscles are doing the work. Don't press your hands against the back of your head—because this will only give you a pain in the neck!

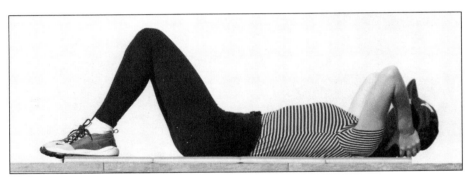

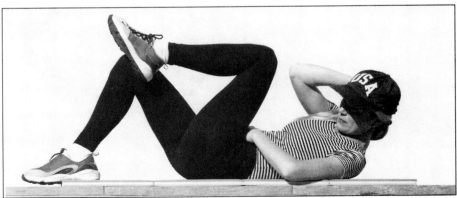

D) Reverse Crunches

1. Your back is flat on the floor. Legs are raised with the knees bent at 45 degrees so that your thighs are perpendicular to the floor. Your arms are along your sides with palms down.

2. Using your abdominal muscles, lift your knees toward your chest, which will also raise the pelvis. Continue the motion until your tailbone comes off the ground. Don't arch your back.
3. Lower your legs to the starting point and repeat.

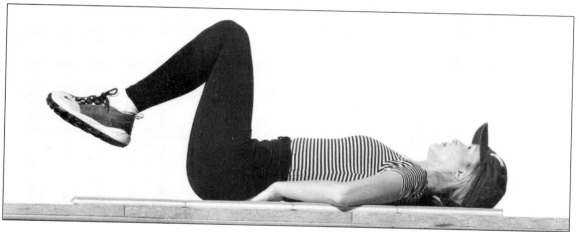

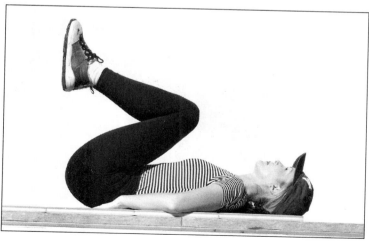

E) Power Pumps

1. Lie flat on the floor with knees bent. Place arms behind your head or cross them on your chest as if you were doing a standard sit-up.
2. Raise your torso off the floor and stop at 45 degrees.
3. Pump up and down just 2 inches either way. Make sure that there is continuous tension on the abdomen.

Pregnancy and giving birth place a tremendous strain on your joints, causing some of them to loosen. In order to return to their normal capacity, these exercises should be performed on a regular basis to prevent any weakening of the tendons that hold the joints in place.

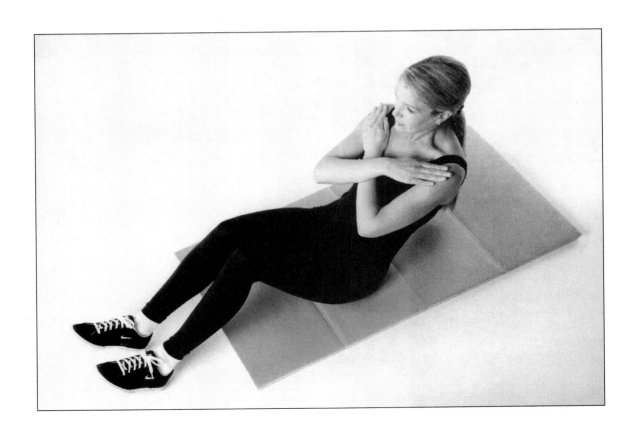

F) Pikes

1. Lie flat on the floor. Knees are slightly bent, heels are resting on the floor. Arms are straight at your sides. Your head and upper shoulders should be slightly elevated off the floor.

2. Bring your knees and chest together by tensing the abdominal muscles, while reaching your hands toward your feet.

3. Return to starting position and repeat.

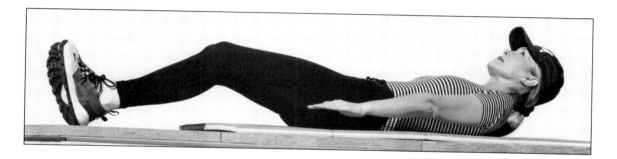

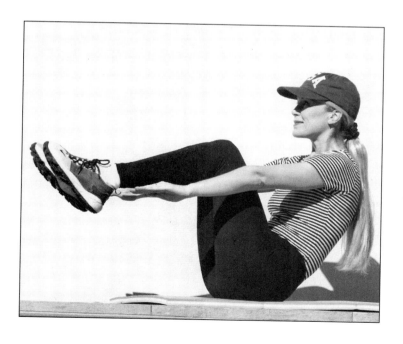

Although I'm not a therapist, I've seen many of my clients become better able to handle pressure and tension after beginning my exercise program. And due to this, I believe many of them have virtually eliminated the effects of postpartum depression. I suppose there's something about "just doing it" that keeps your brain cells positive and up!

G) Alternate Pikes

1. Lie flat on the floor. Knees are slightly bent, heels are resting on the floor. Arms are straight at your sides. Your head and upper shoulders should be slightly elevated off the floor.
2. Bring up your right knee and twist your left shoulder toward it, reaching your hands straight out to the right. Lower to starting position.
3. Bring up your left knee and twist your right shoulder toward it, reaching your hands straight out to the left. Lower to starting position.
4. Repeat from step #2.

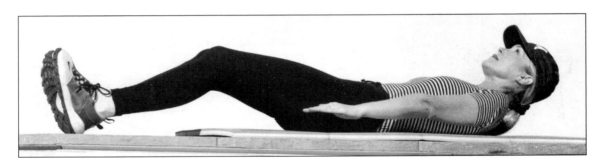

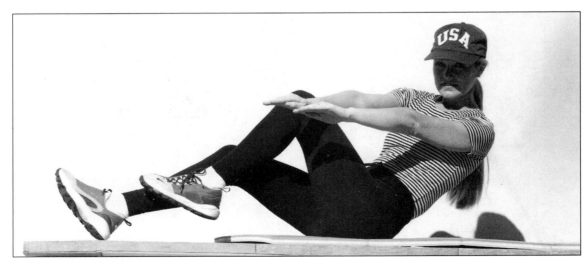

H) Scissors

1. Lie flat on your back. Hands are underneath your tailbone. Legs are straight with heels elevated 6 inches off the floor. Feet are flexed.

2. Spread your legs out to a 45-degree angle. Then bring the feet together. Make sure the heels stay 6 inches off the floor.

3. Return legs to 45-degree angle and repeat: in and out.

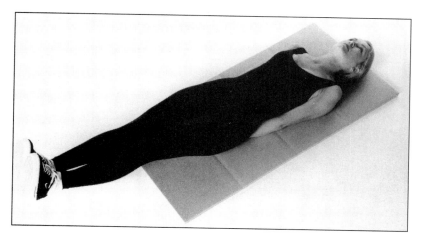

Right now you may feel like collapsing, but don't. You must "cool down" your muscles in order to prevent injury and get the maximum results from your workout.

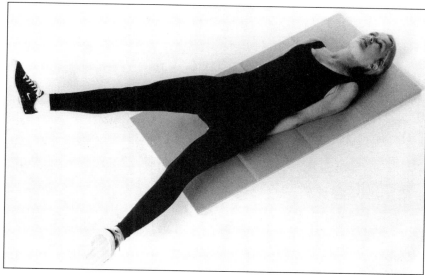

I) Crosses

1. Lie flat on your back. Hands are underneath your tailbone. Legs are spread out to a 45-degree angle with heels elevated 6 inches off the floor.

2. Bring your legs together and cross your left leg over your right. Return them to the 45-degree angle. Make sure the heels stay 6 inches off the floor.

3. Now bring your legs together and cross your right leg over your left. Return them to the 45-degree angle and repeat from step #2.

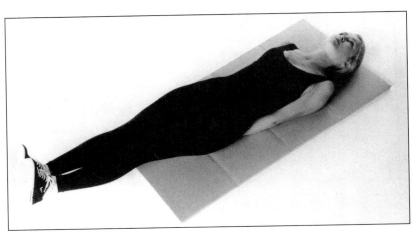

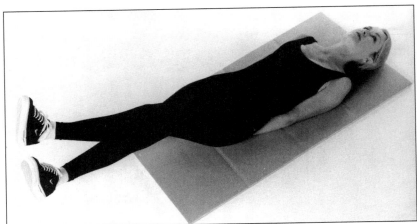

J) Dead Man's Kick

1. Lie flat on your back. Hands are underneath your tailbone. Legs are straight with heels elevated 12 inches off the floor.
2. Lower your right leg straight down until your heel is 6 inches off the floor. Be sure that your lower back remains on the floor.
3. Raise the right leg back to the starting position.
4. Lower your left leg straight down until your heel is 6 inches off the floor.
5. Raise the left leg back to the starting position and repeat.

> If at the end of your workout you find yourself completely fatigued, just totally drained, then you've been exercising a bit too strenuously. Don't worry about it. Take it a bit easier the next time. After exercising you should experience a clear sense of exhilaration, not exhaustion.

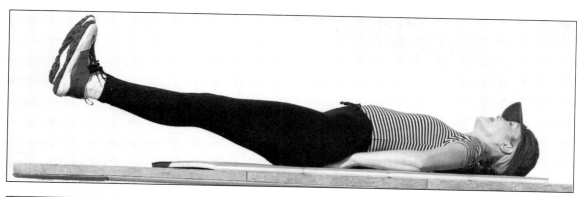

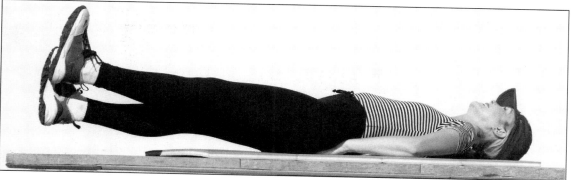

The Pre-Pregnancy Workout

Congratulations. But you haven't reached the end of the road—only the beginning. What lies ahead is years of good health and vitality. You might have guessed by now that the Post-Pregnancy Workout is also the Pre-Pregnancy Workout. Staying with the exercise program will absolutely guarantee that after having your next child, you will bounce back into shape at supersonic speed, just like Demi, Maria, Patty, and Tatum have.

There is no reason why many of these routines cannot be performed during pregnancy as well. However, I caution you to consult a qualified physician, preferably a licensed Ob/Gyn, before choosing to continue exercising during the months you're expecting. Only a doctor can best advise you about how challenging your regimen should be while you're carrying a child, since every woman is different and has special needs.

About the Authors

Rob Parr is a renowned personal trainer who has worked with celebrity clients such as Demi Moore, Bruce Willis, Sharon Stone, John McEnroe, Tatum O'Neal, Maria Shriver, Alicia Silverstone, Whoopi Goldberg and Stevie Nicks. Rob is the trainer responsible for the highly publicized reshaping of Madonna. Rob trained Madonna for four years, getting her in top shape for her first two world tours, the feature film *Dick Tracy* and countless videos.

Raised in Santa Monica, California, Rob Parr attended CalPoly at San Luis Obispo on a baseball scholarship and studied exercise physiology. In his first year, he was drafted by Oakland, but waited until 1980 to sign with the San Francisco Giants. Rob launched his own personal style of fitness training after his career with the Giants ended.

His much sought-after fitness workouts take him around the world as he exclusively designs them for the lifestyles and interests of his clients. He lives in Los Angeles with his wife, Debra, and his three children, Jordan, Chandler and Hunter.

David A. Rudnitsky is a professional screenwriter for film and television. Recently he coauthored Tammy Faye Bakker's autobiography for Random House. In addition, Mr. Rudnitsky has written six other books to date. Among them, in the field of self-help psychology: *Love Codes; 1001 Ways You Reveal Your Personality* and *1001 MORE Ways You Reveal Your Personality* plus *Parents Who Stay Lovers.*

He has also written the following humorous titles: *The Joy of Depression* as well as *Men Who Hate Themselves—And the Women Who Agree with Them.*

Mr. Rudnitsky's books have broad international appeal and have appeared in more than twenty countries, including France, England, Brazil, Japan, Germany, Israel and Turkey. Additionally, they have been excerpted or serialized in hundreds of newspapers and magazines, including *Cosmopolitan, Mademoiselle, Playboy, Penthouse, People, Us, High Times, Self, Seventeen, American Way* and *Working Woman.* They have been featured on *Oprah, Live with Regis & Kathy Lee, Geraldo,* Comedy Central, *Larry King Live* and *Donahue.*

Mr. Rudnitsky has been a senior creative force at some of America's most prestigious advertising agencies, including Saatchi and Saatchi, Lintas Worldwide, Young & Rubicam and McCann-Erickson, producing commercials for accounts such as Wendy's, Coca-Cola, Levis, Toyota, Hilton Hotels, IBM and American Express. Currently, he is associated with one of the nation's most successful infomercial development companies.

Mr. Rudnitsky divides his time between Los Angeles and New York.